Prolonging Healthful Living with a Fiber-Rich Diet

Hans Fisher

Professor Emeritus, Nutritional Biochemistry, Rutgers University

Author (with Eugene Boe) of

The Rutgers Guide to Lowering Your Cholesterol

This book is dedicated to the memory of
John Francis (Irving) Casey, 1921-2009,
whose ideas, experience and great wit helped
provide the author with the impetus
for writing this volume.

Table of Contents

Introduction

Man has been concerned with his mortality from earliest recorded time. In the oldest surviving epic poem, GILGAMESH, dating from about 2750 BCE, the hero Gilgamesh searches for immortality that, however, always eludes him. Adam and Eve, in the Bible, lose their opportunity for immortality by eating the forbidden fruit from the tree "in the middle of the garden (of Eden)."

In his profound examination of resurrection and eternal life in the Hebrew Bible, Jon Levenson points to the "fountain of life" in Psalm 36:10, and then continues: "The evidence suggests that the Temple (in Jerusalem), too- properly approached and respected- was thought to be an antidote to death, giving a kind of immortality to those who dwell there in innocence, purity, and trust."

Later, explorers searched for the Fountain of Youth, among them Alexander the Great who looked for it in Asia; the Polynesians who located it in Hawaii and of course, Ponce de Leon who followed an Indian tale that located the fountain in Florida.

Toward the end of the 16th century *The Art of Living Long* was published by Luigi Cornaro from Venice. Cornaro had reached the venerable age of 98 and prescribed eating small amounts of food in order to live longer. This book was very popular and has been reprinted many times, as recently again as 2005. The first major scientific advance in longevity research, other than longer life as a result of the successful combating of infectious and, later, metabolic diseases, was the observation in 1935 by Clive M. McKay from Cornell University that caloric restriction (reduced food intake) greatly increased the life span of rats. Since that time similar results have been obtained with other species that have been studied, including, most recently, with primates.

Although no direct evidence exists to suggest that humans would also live longer if they reduced their food intake, it is questionable whether many people would agree to such a regimen that, at least initially, would leave one hungry and dissatisfied.

Enter fiber. A painless way to reduce one's calorie intake is to increase fiber consumption. Fiber provides the bulk needed to induce satiety, a topic that will be discussed in greater detail later in this book. In addition to what may be the most overlooked way to extend our life span, fiber has other attributes that further enhance the promise of better health during our later years. Fiber in the diet has been shown to lower blood cholesterol, to improve the insulin/blood sugar picture in diabetes and epidemiologists have suggested that fiber plays a role in preventing heart disease, diabetes, obesity and colon cancer.

In this text we intend to review the present-day information on fiber: what it is, how it is determined, its physiological and biochemical role in the body, the foods that best provide it and some recipes that incorporate goodly amounts of fiber in tasty dishes.

CHAPTER 1
Food Intake Regulation

The Physiology of Food Intake

As a result of the obesity epidemic afflicting the US and other Western populations, there has been an enormous advance in our understanding of the physiological basis of food intake in man and animals.

Miguel Lopez and associates from the School of Medicine, University of Santiago de Compostela in Spain have recently superbly reviewed this literature in the *Proceedings of the Nutrition Society* (English).

The earlier theories concerning the regulation of food intake were based on the assumption that blood levels of nutrients, glucose (glucostatic hypothesis), fats (lipostatic hypothesis), or amino acids (aminostatic hypothesis) were responsible for signals to the brain that triggered eating or stopping to eat. In the last decade our knowledge of food intake regulation has taken a giant leap forward and we now know that this regulation involves many body organs interacting with the nervous system.

Organs, including the gastrointestinal tract, the thyroid gland, muscle tissue, adipose tissue (fat stores), and the gonads send signals "that inform brain centres of the nutritional, as well as metabolic, status of the animal."

The nervous system associated with the gastrointestinal tract, also known as the enteric nervous system, is involved with all aspects of the digestive processes from chewing the food to defecation.

At least five gut hormones have been identified that play an important role in helping to maintain energy balance in the animal body. The first of these to have been recognized, almost 30 years ago, was **cholecystokinin**, a hormone secreted by the small intestine in response to nutrient intake. The other major hormone of very recent discovery is **ghrelin**. This hormone is synthesized in the stomach, small intestine, colon and cecum. Among other functions, ghrelin "induces positive energy balance...by decreasing fat utilization without markedly changing energy expenditure or locomotor activity." Blood levels of ghrelin are regulated by food intake, rising during fasting and falling after eating. Intravenous injection of ghrelin into healthy people increases food intake.

Several hormones that influence food intake and energy balance are secreted by adipose tissue, a tissue that was at one time believed to be metabolically completely inert and just a storehouse for fat. Two of these hormones are **leptin** and **adiponectin**.

Leptin levels in the blood are highly correlated with the amount of total adipose tissue (body fat). Food restriction suppresses leptin circulation until feeding is restarted. When leptin was first discovered at Rockefeller University it was hoped to be the answer to the obesity crisis in our society. Unfortunately, it was soon discovered that obese people, contrary to expectation, had high circulating levels of leptin, suggesting leptin insensitivity or resistance. Human milk contains leptin and this probably explains why breast-fed babies seldom become obese, because at a certain point, the ingested leptin will suppress appetite and the baby will stop nursing.

Adiponectin is increased following food restriction, and administering the hormone to animals has been shown to reduce body weight gain.

Another pathway in the regulation of food intake, involves the rewarding nature of food, the nervous system and particularly the hypothalamus. Three signaling systems have been recognized in this regard, involving opioids, dopamine and serotonin. These compounds appear to be non-specific in their action on the nervous system by inhibiting not only food intake but also other "rewarding" substances such as alcohol and drugs of abuse. The author of this book discovered that the combination of a dopaminergic and a serotonergic drug was vastly more efficacious in inhibiting alcohol consumption than either drug alone (Alcohol.Clin.Exp.Res.Vol 19, No 1,1995 pp 160-163). The same drug combination, Fen-Phen (fenfluramine and phentermine) enjoyed great weight-loss success until fenfluramine was withdrawn by the Food and Drug Administration because of serious side effects.

It should be clear from this short synopsis that energy regulation in the body is very complex and subject to many interacting pathways. Thus, despite a wealth of interesting leads for the pharmacological treatment of food intake and obesity, we may be well advised to follow some common sense approaches regarding fiber intake as explained next.

Diet Formulation and Food and Calorie Intake

In formulating commercial rations for the production of meat animals such as pigs and poultry, it's been recognized for a very long time that biologically and cost efficient diets must be balanced so as to meet both the animals' calorie as well as their bulk needs. If the calorie needs only are addressed in formulating the diet, there will be an over consumption of food until the bulk/volume needs are also satisfied. Conversely, if the diet is overly rich in bulk/fiber, food intake will stop before an adequate quantity of nutrients has been consumed, a situation that can lead to malnutrition.

Human beings, in the short run, will not respond as precisely as animals to the calorie/bulk balance experience. Our highly developed nervous system and brain is easily influenced by such characteristics of food as taste, smell, texture; attributes that, again in the short haul, can override the physiological balancing phenomenon of calories and bulk. In the long run, however, most of us are sensitive to the calorie/bulk relationship in the same way as are animals.

A definitive experiment that illustrates the interactions among food intake, fiber and caloric density was reported over 50 years ago by researchers at Cornell University. Fred Hill and Leonard Dansky (Poultry Science 33:112-119, 1954) fed young chickens a standard diet for rapid growth that relied on corn meal, a low-fiber cereal, as the main energy source. They then replaced part of the corn meal, in 10% increments, with equivalent amounts of essentially calorie-free oat hulls. The results they obtained are shown in the table:

Modification of Diet	Average Weight (gm)	Food Consumption (gm)	Metabolizable Energy (Kcal)	Protein Consumed (gm)
Control	645	1354	2908	271
+10 oathulls	646	1393	2633	278
+20 oathulls	666	1593	2585	319
+30 oathulls	648	1664	2283	333
+40 oathulls	642	1816	2021	363

After 6 weeks on these diets the average body weight (second column) of all five groups of chickens was very similar, despite large differences in calorie intake (column four).

Column 3 makes the point very succinctly: reduce the caloric density of the diet (by substituting oat hull for corn meal) and food intake is dramatically increased. Yet, despite a 34% increase in food intake, the calorie consumption decreased nevertheless by 30% (2908 vs. 2021 Kcal, column 4). So how explain the similar body weight of all the different groups of animals? Clearly, as the level of fiber (oat hulls) increased, and food consumption also increased, additionally, the efficiency of utilizing the available calories also increased. This is one of the problems encountered by obese people when they reduce their food/calorie intake in an effort to lose weight. Their body machinery adjusts to the reduction by utilizing the consumed food more efficiently. From an evolutionary point of view, this is how early man survived the vicissitudes of food shortages, those who adapted to this greater efficiency survived; yet we, in our world of food plethora, face the opposite problem, plenty of attractive food choices, followed by overeating and obesity.

The fifth and last column in the table brings home another important lesson about the interaction between dietary energy and food consumption. When the calorie density of the diet is changed, as when increasing amounts of fiber (oat hulls) are substituted for corn meal (mostly corn starch), the consumption of other nutrients, as for example protein, is increased as the animal tries to meet its energy needs. This leads to considerable wastage. It is clear from the table that the control group did just fine with its consumption of 271 grams of protein. Thus, the high oat hulls group that consumed 363 grams of protein was wasting 92 grams of protein, or fully one third of its total protein intake. The lesson to be learned is that we must adjust our intake of the other essential nutrients when alterations are made to our calorie consumption.

The importance of fiber in the diet in relation to satiety and the control of food intake was demonstrated also in a study where rats were given a palatable solution containing mannitol, an unabsorbable, slightly sweet soluble fiber. Meal size consumption was reduced in direct proportion to the amount of mannitol in the solution. This reduction was due to the filling of the small intestine and lasted as long as this organ remained filled.

Fiber and the Digestive Process

The human intestine is about 20 to 30 feet in length, depending on the age and size of the individual. The small intestine, the portion connected to the stomach, and the section where most of the digestion and absorption of nutrients takes place, makes up about

80 % of the total length. The large intestine, which includes the colon, is wider in diameter than the small intestine but only about 5 feet long, or 20 % of the total intestinal length. Few of us give serious thought to the marvel that is the anatomy of our digestive tract. Normally when something needs to be propelled through a long tube, say a hose, it needs to be stretched out to permit easy passage. Yet the human intestine is coiled up in our abdominal area and takes up minimal space. So how do food and the products of digestion move through the intestine?

Embedded in the wall of the intestine are nerve endings that are stimulated by pressure against the intestinal wall and that bring about a type of movement called *peristalsis*. Stalsis, in Greek means contraction and peristalsis is a wave of contractions that moves the contents of the intestine along while the intestine itself remains in place. The extent of this type of movement is very dependent on the density or bulkiness of the intestinal content. It takes a relatively small quantity of fiber-rich foods in comparison to highly dense, low-fiber foods to stimulate meaningful peristaltic action. As food passes through the intestine it is mixed with copious amounts of fluid and forms boluses, or balls that are the vehicles that exert the pressure against the intestinal wall that, in turn, stimulate the embedded nerve endings to set up the motion. Low fiber foods generally produce little peristaltic action resulting in a sluggish intestine that has difficulty in producing proper laxation. This can lead to the accumulation of food or products of digestion lodging in the folds of the intestine and serving as the substrate for microorganisms that can produce toxic including carcinogenic compounds. High-fiber foods, on the other hand, will, by virtue of their greater bulk and affinity for liquids, stimulate better laxation and a sharply decreased potential for the intestinal bacterial synthesis of harmful chemicals.

Contrary to the fad that swept the U.S. recently, a low carbohydrate diet makes it difficult to consume an adequate amount of fiber. That is so because fiber is so much a part of grains, fruits and vegetables that it is well nigh impossible to get one's fill of fiber without ingesting reasonably large amounts of carbohydrate-rich foods. As will be discussed later, the type of fiber best suited for stimulating the peristaltic activity of the digestive tract is water insoluble fiber. Cellulose is an important member of this class of fiber. It has great water-absorbing capacity, an attribute that contributes to the volume of intestinal material that exerts pressure and induces the motion leading to proper laxation.

The water soluble fibers, as will be discussed in greater detail later, possess another important property: they slow the absorption of glucose, the main fuel necessary for maintaining proper body function. This characteristic is important in relation to the dietary treatment of diabetes.

Fat and Water in the Context of Proper Nutrition and a Balanced Diet

The importance of specific dietary fat components in the economy of body metabolism has only been recognized within the last three decades.

Quantitatively, the fat group known as triglycerides or triacylglycerides makes up most of the fat found in body tissues and in plant seeds and other plant tissues. This type of fat is composed of two component parts: glycerol, hence the name glycerides, and the signature component—the fatty acids. Each molecule of glycerol, a three carbon compound derived from the 6 carbon sugar glucose, can attach 3 fatty acids unto itself. These fatty acids can all be the same, or all three can be different or 2 may be different and one is the same. Essentially when we speak of fat our concerns generally rest with the nature of the fatty acids. With very rare exceptions, all fatty acids are composed of an even number of carbons and the most important ones, both qualitatively and quantitatively, contain between 14 and about 26 carbons.

Within this group of fatty acids we have several distinct subgroups with different functions and activities. One group that is relatively inert chemically is the group known as saturated fatty acids. These are distinguished by having their carbon atoms surrounded with hydrogen, thus the term "saturated" refers to the fact that the carbons are all attached to hydrogen atoms that saturate all carbon chemical linkages. These fatty acids are usually found in storage sites in the body and also provide insulation in animals that habituate cold climates. Chemically, saturated fatty acids are preferentially utilized by the body in the synthesis of cholesterol. From this vantage point it is advisable to limit one's intake of saturated fatty acids (or triglycerides). The so called tropical fats, coconut oil, cocoa butter, palm oil and palm kernel oil are fully saturated and may also, preferentially, contribute to greater cholesterol synthesis in the body.

The chemical removal of two hydrogen bonds from between two adjacent carbons leads to the creation of a double bond. Since every carbon must, for chemical stability, be surrounded by four bonds, usually hydrogen, the removal of two hydrogen bonds creates a doubling up of bonds between the adjacent carbons. This type of fatty acid with a double bond is chemically less stable but also more chemically reactive. Thus, a fatty acid with a double bond may play a role in helping the body get rid of excess cholesterol.

The most prevalent single double bond fatty acid is called oleic acid and is present in high concentrations in olive oil. Oleic acid has 18 carbons and one double bond.

Fatty acids with two or more double bonds cannot be synthesized by the body and must be supplied with our food. For this reason fatty acids with two and three double bonds are also referred to as "essential" fatty acids. The most common fatty acid with two double bonds is linoleic acid, an 18 carbon fatty acid widely present in seed oils including, corn, cottonseed, soybean, safflower and sunflower among others. Fatty acids with three double bonds include linolenic acid an 18 carbon fatty acid found in soybean oil in small amounts and in larger amounts in linseed oil. Fatty acids with 4-6 double bonds are found in many fish oils and a few esoteric plant sources.

Two terms are usually used to describe the unsaturated fatty acids that are of metabolic significance: omega 3 and omega 6 fatty acids. These terms refer to the location of the first double bond along the carbon chain of the fatty acid. An omega 3 double bond occurs between carbons 3 and 4 counting from the left end, whereas an omega 6 double bond occurs between carbons 6 and 7 also counting from the left hand side of the molecule.

Both types of fatty acid are essential and fulfill important physiological functions in the body. They are used in the synthesis of compounds known as prostaglandins, prostacyclins and thromboxane, among others. These compounds have hormonal properties that help in the regulation of blood pressure, blood clotting and other functions.

Water is probably the most neglected among the nutrients that are essential for life. It is somehow taken for granted that we fulfill our water needs through thirst-driven drinking. Unfortunately that is not always the case. To begin at the beginning, water constitutes 72 % of the fat free body, not only in human beings but in all animals. This interesting fact points to a relationship between water and fat in the composition of the body. If we assume an average fat content of 18% for a man, this translates to a water content for that individual of 59%. Women, who generally have somewhat more body fat, consequently have somewhat less body water.

The water requirement of people living and working in a temperate climate where they do not sweat, normally is about 1 gram or milliliter for every kilocalorie of energy expenditure. Thus a person with a maintenance energy need of 2000 kilocalories requires about 2000 grams or 2 liters of water.

We derive our water needs from three sources: drinking liquids is generally the most important source, followed by water that is part of the foods we consume. Many fruits and vegetables are very high in water content and can thus contribute significantly to our overall water intake. Lastly, there is a category called metabolic water. This is the water produced from the chemical reactions that carbohydrates, fats and proteins undergo during their metabolism in the body. As these nutrients are converted into the energy needed to run the body machinery including the pumping of the heart, the filtration processes of the kidneys, the contractions of the muscles during every movement that we make, a small but meaningful amount of water is formed.

The excretory routes of water occur by way of four organs: the lungs, during breathing exhalation; the skin, through perspiration, the intestine as part of the fecal matter we excrete and the kidneys that produce the urine that contains waste products of metabolism, mostly from protein. Depending on the rate of our activity and the altitude where we live, the amount of water lost through the lungs can amount to several 100 milliliters per day. The 1952 British Expedition to climb Mount Everest failed because the climbers failed to take into account the very low oxygen pressure at the very high altitudes that led to rapid breathing and great water loss. The climbers drunk about a pint a day and it was later calculated that they needed 5-7 pints.

We lose between 100 and 600 milliliters of water a day through what is known as "insensible" perspiration; that is, perspiration not related to sweating. With heavy activity or high environmental temperature, sweating may add considerably to the water loss through the skin.

Water loss through the intestine is generally minimal but can jump to a high volume if a gastrointestinal infection leads to severe diarrhea such as in cholera where water replacement is uppermost on the treatment agenda. Kidney water loss can vary from as little as 300 milliliters to as much as 7 liters depending upon the amount of water consumed.

Unfortunately, thirst does not always help us regulate our water intake in sufficient amounts   A very high protein intake requires more water to help with the elimination of the products of its metabolism and kidney stones may often be prevented with adequate water consumption.

CHAPTER 2
How we Define, Classify and Analyze Fiber?

My American Heritage Dictionary of the English Language cites 9 definitions under the heading fiber. The first and most universal one states that fiber is "any slender, elongated structure; a filament or strand." Definition 2 is the one that comes closest to our nutritional concept: according to this definition, fiber is "one of the elongated, thick-walled cells that give strength and support to plant tissue."

A more appropriate definition was coined by Trowell who explained *dietary fiber* as "the skeletal remains of plant cells that are resistant to digestion by enzymes of man." Another, more recently added term, is *functional fiber*, which refers to fiber that shows beneficial action in people.

In the digestive tract fiber exhibits several physico-chemical properties. These include water-holding capacity, adsorptive function, cation-exchange and bacterial fermentation. It is these properties that impart to dietary fiber its clinical significance.

Until recently fibers were further subdivided into two groups, water *soluble* and water insoluble. The water soluble fibers include pectins, gums, and mucilages and they are separated out from such insoluble fibers as cellulose and lignin because of their greater binding or trapping capacity due to gelling when in contact with water. This attribute, also referred to as viscosity, inhibits the absorption of dietary food cholesterol and even saturated fatty acids from within the gastrointestinal mass. The soluble fibers are also more readily attacked by bacteria in the large intestine where they can be metabolized into the so-called volatile fatty acids, acetic, propionic and butyric acid. The water insoluble fibers such as cellulose and lignin were once considered primarily beneficial as bulk formers and aids to laxation. But recent findings show that both soluble and insoluble fibers possess this property. Similarly, the trapping properties of soluble fibers have also been found to a lesser degree in insoluble fiber. Thus it has been suggested to use the terms *viscous* and *nonfermentable* in place of soluble and insoluble.

With the exception of lignin, a small, low molecular weight polymer, the other common sources of fiber are all carbohydrates, which belong to the family of polysaccharides (poly-many; saccharides-sugars). Cellulose is chemically the simplest of the fibers, its composition consists of an unbranched chain containing about 3000 glucose units. The hemicelluloses are not at all related to cellulose yet the name, which dates back to 1891, has been retained. These carbohydrates are more complex and contain mixtures of 5- and 6-carbon sugars that exhibit considerable branching.

Pectins are present in relatively large amounts in citrus fruit rind and sugar beet pulp (30 %), apple skin (15%), and tomatoes(21%). Pectins contain a mix of galacturonic acid, galactose, arabinose and xylose among other sugars. They are particularly important because of their gelling properties. This characteristic also makes them useful from a dietary health perspective as will be discussed later.

Plant gums and mucilages come from different parts of the plant than do the pectins and hemicelluloses. The former often are found at the site of an injury to a plant and constitute a material that oozes from that injury. Mucilages are found in seeds where they seem to serve as a storage vehicle for moisture to prevent the drying out of the seed. Chemically, both groups represent very complex polysaccharide structures that are highly branched and composed of uronic acid (a sugar acid) residues in combination with several sugars.

Another water- soluble fiber, glucomannan, is derived from the konjac root. Konjac is a perennial plant found mostly in Asia and long cultivated in Japan. About 30% of the dry material in the root consists of glucomannan, the remaining 70% is starch. Glucomannan has strong bulking properties and probably also prevents dietary cholesterol absorption.

The different components of what we normally define as fiber are to be found in all parts of the plant, including root, stem, leaf, fruit and seed. The proportions depend on the maturity of the plant, with greater lignin and insoluble fiber content occurring as the plant becomes older and more mature. Generally, for human consumption, we tend to eat most parts of plants, with the exception of the seeds, when the plant it still relatively immature so that lignification will be low and the soluble fiber content will be comparatively higher.

High fiber diets, because of the bulkiness that they provide, produce greater satiety in the person consuming them than a low fiber diet. Thus, to match the same volume of food that a high fiber diet contributes, more calories of a low fiber diet will have to be ingested to provide a similar sense of fullness or satiety.

An interesting point has been raised about the protein that is associated with the plant cell wall or that is found in the feces as indigestible from other origins. Some researchers make a strong case for including indigestible protein with the term "fiber" because, these folks say, the protein has chemically reactive groups that may be important in the physiological role that fiber plays. This might involve, for instance, the binding effect of fiber on certain fat components of the diet.

The analysis for fiber is very intricate as might be expected from the chemical complexity of the different structures from which it is composed. To this day we still use a very old method to determine what is generally referred to as *crude fiber*. Then, if greater specificity is desired, more specialized procedures are used to determine the content of pectin, gums or other components.

The crude fiber determination involves the serial extraction of a food sample to remove, first, the fat, then the protein and carbohydrate. The fat is usually extracted from an air-dried sample with either ether or petroleum ether. This extraction is followed by boiling the residue in sulfuric acid, followed by filtering and washing with hot water. Next, the residue from the acid extraction is boiled with sodium hydroxide, a strong alkaline solution, followed by filtering, washing with hot acid, hot water and alcohol. The resulting residue is dried and weighed. It is then placed in a muffle furnace set at 600ºC and ashed. The ash residue is weighed and the crude fiber constitutes the difference between the weight prior to ashing and following ashing.

CHAPTER 3

Health-related Functions of Fiber-Cholesterol, Atherosclerosis and Heart Disease

The person largely credited with calling public attention to the importance of fiber in our diet is Denis Burkitt, a British surgeon who spent many years in Uganda and while there, discovered the disease known as Burkitt's Lymphoma. When he returned from Africa in the late 1960's he began advocating high fiber diets because African natives who consumed such diets had a much lower incidence of gastrointestinal diseases and disorders than Europeans.

About the time that Burkitt started publicizing the apparent importance of fiber in the diet an estimate of dietary fiber consumption in 38 countries was calculated from food disappearance tables collected by the Food and Agricultural Organization (FAO), a body of the United Nations. Although no data are given for African nations, there are very large differences in fiber consumption among those countries that are listed. Bulgaria leads among these 38 countries with an estimated intake of 16.1 grams/day of crude fiber. Also showing high fiber intakes were Romania, Mexico, Greece and Portugal. Sweden, Switzerland, Finland the United Kingdom, Australia and the United States are on the other end of the scale, with only 5-6 grams of crude fiber consumed per day.

Calculations have also been reported on the changes in crude fiber consumption in the US between 1909 and 1975. According to these figures there was a 28 % decrease in fiber consumption between 1909 and 1959 but the values have remained steady since then. The consumption of whole grains as a source of fiber is low in the U.S. It is estimated that " fewer than 1 in 10 adults eat three servings of whole grains a day. And about 4 out of 10 eat none."

Burkitt, was not the first to have noted a possible relationship between dietary fiber and other human diseases. In 1960, Ancel Keys, a renowned physiologist on the faculty of the University of Minnesota, suggested that fiber, such as pectin, was probably responsible for the significantly lower blood cholesterol levels of Italian men from Naples compared to men from Minnesota. In a follow-up experiment Keys observed a reduction in blood cholesterol within 3 weeks among middle-aged men given a pectin supplement compared to others who got cellulose. In these studies the diet always provided cholesterol from various food sources.

In 1963, my research group at Rutgers University, working with male and female chickens as experimental animals, tested Army C rations for their atherogenic (heart disease causing) properties. Following the Korean War in the 50's, there was concern that the Army C rations might have contributed to the considerable degree of fatty deposits found in the major blood vessels of American soldiers who had been killed in combat and who were autopsied. The Quartermaster Corps contracted with us to check into this question. Most surprisingly, because the C Rations contained meat, eggs and milk products, we observed just the opposite results of what had been anticipated. The birds on the C Rations had significantly less atherosclerotic involvement than the controls on an ordinary, cholesterol-free, poultry ration. We conjectured, in the light of Keys' findings that some component of the C Ration was providing protection against the dietary cholesterol and the saturated fat. Indeed, it turned out that the sugar beet pulp that we had added to the Army Rations to help absorb moisture and thus make the mix more palatable to the chickens had provided 3-4% pectin as a percentage of the total diet.

Armed with this unexpected information, we set up a new experiment in which one group of cockerels was fed 5% pectin and a control group was given 5% cellulose. The diet was a standard, corn-soybean ration free of animal products, cholesterol and saturated fats. After 18 months, when the birds were sacrificed we found that the pectin had prevented the onset of atherosclerosis (the accumulation of fatty deposits in major blood vessels), even on the diet that was free of cholesterol. Moreover, the pectin-fed cockerels excreted in their feces three-times as much fat and twice-as much cholesterol as the controls that had received cellulose. These findings were extended to other animal species, rabbits and pigs, among others. We also experimented with additional sources of soluble fiber. Besides pectin, carrageenan (a seaweed extract), guar gum, scleroglucan (a natural polymer produced by fermentation), barley and oat hulls all have strong cholesterol-lowering properties when added to cholesterol-containing diets.

As shown in the results of the fecal analyses discussed in the last paragraph, these fiber sources appear to have a propensity to bind either directly to cholesterol or to bile acids(bile acids are breakdown products from cholesterol) and thus help reduce the absorption or re-absorption of cholesterol from the digestive tract.

In 1982 another strong bit of evidence concerning the importance of dietary fiber in relation to heart disease was published from the Netherlands. Kromhout and associates from the State University of Leiden reported on a 10-year mortality examination of deaths in the town of Zutphen. They observed that the mortality from heart disease was four times higher in men on the lowest fiber intake compared to men on the highest intake. Deaths from cancer and all other causes were also about three times higher on the low fiber intake compared to deaths on the high fiber diets. These researchers concluded that "A diet containing at least 37 grams dietary fibre per day may be protective against chronic diseases in Western societies."

The Zutphen population was recently re-visited in relation to the incidence of coronary heart disease and fiber intake(June 2008). The study showed that "recent dietary fiber intake was inversely associated with coronary heart disease and all-cause mortality risk."

An increased intake of every 10 g of recent dietary fiber per day lowered heart disease mortality by 17 % and all-cause mortality by 9 %. The source of dietary fiber did not seem to affect the findings.

It has long been accepted as a given that high blood cholesterol levels constitute an important risk factor for heart disease. Although we have important drugs available today to lower blood cholesterol, particularly the group of drugs known as statins, several water-soluble sources of fiber, including pectin, guar gum, psyllium and oat bran, among others, also have strong blood cholesterol-lowering properties. A recent review of fourteen studies in which gluco-mannan was given to human subjects under well-controlled conditions also showed that this fiber source beneficially affected total cholesterol, LDLcholesterol, triglycerides, body weight and fasting blood glucose but not HDLcholesterol or blood pressure. The statins lower blood cholesterol by interfering with its synthesis in many body tissues but particularly the liver. The group of fibers just listed lower blood cholesterol by preventing cholesterol absorption from food, by binding some saturated fats that serve as major precursors for cholesterol synthesis, and by binding and eliminating in the feces bile salts that are derived from cholesterol and therefore cause greater conversion in the liver of cholesterol to bile salts to make up for those lost to binding in the intestines.

Since pure pectin has been reported by us and others as an effective cholesterol-lowering fiber, it was of special interest to note that a food-source of pectin was equally effective. In this study healthy individuals were given between 4 and 9 grams of pectin per day by ingesting 2-3 apples daily. After one month there were significant reductions in the subjects' blood cholesterol.

Cholesterol circulates in the blood as part of chemical entities called lipoproteins. These compounds contain protein and fatty acids. One type of cholesterol-containing lipoprotein, the LDL or low-density lipoprotein, is considered bad for us because it cannot easily be eliminated from the body and can cause obstruction of blood vessels leading to heart attacks, particularly in the coronary or heart arteries. The other major type of cholesterol-containing lipoprotein, the HDL or high-density lipoprotein, is beneficial because it helps cholesterol to get eliminated when in excess and it is less likely to settle out and obstruct blood flow in the arteries of the body. In a major recent study it was shown that cereals that were enriched with psyllium not only lowered total blood cholesterol but specifically reduced only the LDL-bound cholesterol without affecting the level of HDL-bound cholesterol in people with mild to moderately elevated blood cholesterol levels.

Not only has cholesterol lowering been reported as a result of a higher intake of dietary fiber, but newer technologies available for measuring the progression of atherosclerosis have also shown important improvement from higher fiber consumption. The Cardiovascular Nutrition Laboratory at Tufts University studied "the association between intakes of total fiber from different dietary sources and progression of coronary-artery artherosclerosis among women with established coronary artery disease." Among 229 postmenopausal women, those with fiber intakes greater than 3 grams/ 1000 kcalories of cereal fiber or more than 6 servings of whole grains per week had smaller declines in minimum coronary artery diameter. Stated another way, a higher intake of cereal fiber, but not fruit and vegetable fiber, showed less progression in percent stenosis (blockage) in coronary arteries.

In a recent review of seven studies comparing cereal fiber intake to heart disease incidence, those who ate two and a half servings of whole grains per day had a 21 percent lower risk of developing heart disease than did people who consumed only a fifth of a serving.

Given the positive effects of whole grain fiber in relation to heart disease, it is interesting to note a very recent study among approximately 29,000 female US Health Professionals free of cardiovascular disease, cancer or hypertension. "Higher whole grain intake was associated with a reduced risk of hypertension in middle-aged and older women…"

A similar finding in men from the Health Professionals Follow-Up Study that evaluated 51,529 men ages 40 to 75 showed "an independent inverse association between intake of whole grains and incident hypertension in men. Bran may play an important role in this association."

Hypertension is one of the major risk factors for heart disease.

Equally impressive are the results of a study with both men and women from the Keck School of

Medicine at the University of Southern California, Los Angeles. The researchers, whose participants were free of heart disease, measured the intima-media thickness of the common carotid arteries ultrasonographically at the start of the study and at two subsequent periods. There was a statistically significant inverse relationship between the progression of intima thickness of the carotids and consumption of viscous fiber, particularly pectin. Blood lipids were also measured and were similarly lowered by increased intake of fiber. The authors suggested that the protection afforded by fiber intake against intima-media thickness progression may well be mediated by the lowered blood lipids.

An epidemiological study from Marseille, France, with 2532 men and 3429 women showed that "(T)he highest total dietary fiber and non-soluble dietary fiber intakes were associated with a significantly (P<0.05) lower risk of overweight...blood pressure..cholesterol, triacylglycerols (triglycerides) and homocysteine." Interestingly, in this survey study soluble dietary fiber was less efficacious than the non-soluble fibers. Non-the-less there was no doubt that dietary fiber offered a protective role against cardiovascular disease.

Finally, a recent case study report from Unity Hospital in Rochester, NY provides very strong further evidence for the importance of fiber in the diet. A healthy 51-year-old man, non-smoker, physically active, with no evidence of heart disease, hypertension or diabetes decided to go on the low-carbohydrate Atkins diet because his weight had started to increase from 63 to 67 kg. After one month on the Atkins diet his total and LDLcholesterol showed a sharp increase while his body weight had decreased to 64 kg. A year and a half later he suffered from erectile dysfunction, his cholesterol had decreased modestly but his triglycerides had increased markedly. A half year later angiography showed a "critical stenosis…of the left anterior descending coronary artery, which was treated with a drug-eluting stent." He stopped the Atkins diet and started on a low-fat, high fiber diet.. Two month later the patient weighed 62 kg, cholesterol levels were back to normal, the erectile dysfunction had stopped and he had no chest pains.

CHAPTER 4
Health-related Functions of Fiber-Diabetes

In January 2007 the Department of Health and Mental Hygiene of the City of New York released a study that showed that one in eight adults in the city suffered from diabetes. Over 90% of these people had Type 2 diabetes, a type that is closely related to obesity. Both diabetes and obesity are among the worst public health problems in the Western World today.

Not long after the discovery of a beneficial effect of certain fibers on cholesterol metabolism, research clinicians in the U.S and in Great Britain noted marked improvements in diabetic patients when they were given high-carbohydrate, high-fiber diets. James Anderson, at the University of Kentucky, noted initially that high carbohydrate- low fat diets improved sensitivity to insulin and improved glucose metabolism. In the mid-70's Anderson and his group began to include increased amounts of fiber in the form of fiber-rich foods into the high-carbohydrate, low-fat diets. With these diets they observed lower insulin requirements, and lower blood glucose, cholesterol and triglyceride values in diabetic patients.

About the same time that these observations were being recorded in the U.S., David Jenkins and co-workers in England and later Canada obtained similar positive results in diabetic patients given high-carbohydrate, high-fiber diets. In one study, 10 men were given a high-fiber diet, mostly from cereals and in 9 of the men a drug treatment could be completely withdrawn or the insulin dose reduced.

Unlike Anderson, Jenkins next turned his attention to using purified fiber supplements with his patients. In a two-pronged study he asked one group of diabetic patients to supplement their home diets with 25 grams of guar gum daily while a second group was given the same amount of this soluble, gel-forming fiber in their metabolic ward diet. The measure of success from the guar gum ingestion was the significant lowering of urinary glucose excretion by

46% and 54% for the two groups of diabetics, respectively. Jenkins helped develop a bread that he called guar crispbread that made the incorporation of guar into a diet for diabetics much easier than having to mix it into various food items like soup, fruit juices or cereals. The crispbread contained about 1 gram of guar per slice and patients consumed between 14 and 25 slices per day in place of regular bread slices.

Other fiber sources have also been shown effective in the treatment of diabetes in patients. In Sweden, a group of men suffering from non-insulin-dependent diabetes (type 2) benefited from 5 grams daily of a sodium alginate supplement to their diet. This is an isolate from algae that contains 75 % soluble fiber. The fiber ingestion resulted in a reduced rise in blood glucose and serum insulin following a meal. The fiber was shown to slow down gastric emptying which was held to be responsible for the beneficial effects on blood sugar and insulin.

Another gum that has also been shown to slow gastric emptying in animals, xanthan gum, has also been shown to reduce blood glucose following a meal. It also reduced cholesterol, particularly the LDL fraction.

In a prisoner population of diabetics in Japan, a high-fiber preparation made up of boiled rice with barley "Mugimeshi," produced dramatic improvements in their diabetic status such that 5 of 18 prisoners treated with insulin and 17 of 34 treated with oral hypoglycemic agents were able to discontinue their drug treatment and maintain good metabolic control.

In South Korea medical researchers reported successful results from a diet enriched with Goami No. 2, a fiber-rich rice, given to obese and non-obese subjects prone for type 2 diabetes. The fiber-rich Goami No. 2 rice significantly lowered body weight in both obese and non-obese people, and also significantly lowered serum triglycerides, total and low density lipoprotein cholesterol, as well as C-peptide.

Another recent study with a new dietary fiber called FBCx was carried out over 3 months in a carefully controlled trial with obese patients with type 2 diabetes. The controls continued to gain weight during the study while those on the fiber diet maintained their starting weight. Total cholesterol decreased 8% in the fiber group while the controls showed a small but significant increase in cholesterol. Adiponectin, a hormone produced by fat cells that suppresses type 2 diabetes, was increased in the fiber group but significantly decreased in the controls. Thus, FBCx appears suitable for incorporation into a diabetes management program.

An important observation was recently reported from the Harvard School of Public Health relating the risk of diabetes during pregnancy to the pre-pregnancy dietary fiber intake. The data were taken from among over 13,000 eligible women who are part of a large, ongoing, Nurses Health Study II. "After adjustment for age, parity, prepregnancy Body Mass Index…dietary total fiber and cereal and fruit fiber were strongly associated with GDM (pregnancy diabetes) risk." The risk of diabetes decreased by 26% with every increase of 10 grams daily in fiber.

The amount of fiber consumed has also recently been reported to relate to periodontitis, or serious gum disease in men. It has been known for some time that diabetes increases the risk of periodontitis, thus in a study from McMaster University in Canada, it was ascertained that men in the highest fiber intake group had a 23% lower risk of getting this potentially serious dental disease that can affect the body in other negative ways including leading to heart attack.

Very interestingly, the Tufts University Research Center on Aging recently reported a relationship between age-related macular degeneration and the carbohydrate component of the diet. The researchers found that carbohydrate-rich foods with a high glycemic index, an indicator of the diet's potential to raise blood sugar levels, was strongly associated with the eye disorder. This means that foods high in simple carbohydrates such as sugar are metabolized rapidly whereas complex carbohydrates, those that are rich in fiber, are metabolized and broken down slowly. This is the same pattern observed for the development of diabetes, cardiovascular disease and possibly some types of cancer.

A recent review of nutritional guidelines for diabetics and compliance with them showed that people with diabetes, in many countries, fall considerably short in eating appropriate diets. In general these diabetics consume more fat and saturated fat than non-diabetics and their carbohydrate and presumably their fiber intake as well, falls below the recommended levels. Except for an intensive intervention program that the author of the review stated to be difficult to achieve, three-monthly dietary counseling sessions did not improve the patients' adherence to a recommended dietary regimen for diabetes. By contrast, Anderson at Kentucky has for many years operated a diabetes support program that features HCF or High-Carbohydrate, High-Fiber diets. Participants purchase a User's Guide and A Professional Guide is available for clinical personnel to help guide patients with their diet regimens.

A recent study from the Department of Medicine at George Washington University showed that a low-fat, vegan diet that supplied considerable dietary fiber was as readily acceptable as a more conventional diabetic diet in which the patients consumed only about half the amount of fiber(26 g vs 14 g).

The evidence for a preventive as well as therapeutic effect of high fiber diets for diabetics, accumulated over the last 30 years is very strong, indeed!

CHAPTER 5

Health-related Functions of Fiber-Disorders of the Lower Digestive Tract

As mentioned at the beginning of Chapter 3, Denis Burkitt, the surgeon who worked in Africa for many years, upon returning to England in the mid 1960's, suggested that gastrointestinal disorders among Europeans and Americans, ranging from constipation to colon cancer, appeared to be the result of low fiber consumption. Africans, by comparison, had a very low incidence of these diseases or disorders.

Some of the interesting information observed in comparing people who normally consumed a high fiber diet with Americans or Europeans eating low fiber diets included the finding that the former had daily stool weights of 500 grams compared to only 100 grams for the latter. Most of the difference in weight consists of water which makes the stools softer, easier to pass and much less likely to cause straining of the large intestine that so often leads to outpouchings in the colon called diverticula.

Another important difference resulting from high versus low fiber intake is the time it takes for food to pass from mouth to the anus. This is called the transit time. African natives are reported to have transit times of about 30 hours compared to transit times for Europeans or Americans of 48 hours or more. A prolonged transit time has been found in patients with diverticular disease.

Before turning our attention to diverticular disease let us briefly consider constipation as an important precursor problem. That constipation is due to the consumption of highly refined, low fiber diets is beyond question. Although at one time it was believed that a sedentary lifestyle and inattention to the call of nature were possible causes of constipation, direct experimentation with diets providing more fiber put such beliefs to rest. In one telling study adult subjects were switched from a diet that included 450 grams of white bread to one that included the same amount of whole grain bread. This dietary change resulted in a decreased food transit time from 28 to 19 hours, an increase in the daily dry fecal matter voided from 29 to 41 grams and an increase in bowel movement frequency from 1 to 1.6 times per day. During World War II it was observed in Ireland that the sale of Epsom salt as a laxative fell by several tons a month when whole-grain bread was the only bread available.

Diverticular disease refers to two conditions: diverticulosis, which involves having outpouchings in the colon that are called diverticula, and diverticulitis, a condition in which the diverticula become inflamed or infected. Men are more prone to these disorders than women and by age 60, it is estimated that 50 % of the American population is subject to these disorders. Between about 1920 and 1970 it was accepted medical practice to treat diverticular disease with a low fiber diet. Today it is well established that a high fiber diet is the appropriate treatment of choice. A diet high in wheat bran was shown very effective over 30 years ago. Today, the treatment recommended consists of a high fiber diet, which, if necessary, might include taking a fiber supplement in addition to high fiber foods. The term "roughage" was at one time used to describe fiber in the diet with the mistaken notion that fiber was abrasive and caused inflammation of the digestive tract. In point of fact it has been found that less mucus appears to be formed and eliminated in the feces on a high, as compared to a low fiber diet.

Two additional reports further strengthen the case for a high fiber diet to prevent or treat gastrointestinal disease. Broadribb from Oxford reported on a carefully controlled trial in which 18 patients with diverticular disease were given either a high-fiber, wheat bran-containing diet or the same diet with wheat flour but no bran. There was a significant effect in obtaining relief on the high-fiber diet compared to the low-fiber diet and the improvement increased over the duration of the trial. In the second study, 26 patients with irritable bowel syndrome were also given either a wheat bran supplement or none. By six weeks on the high-fiber diet there was significant improvement in symptoms on the high- versus the low-fiber diet and there was objective evidence in the patients on the high-fiber diet of a significantly reduced rate of colon motor activity.

Comparison of the incidence of appendicitis between white and black populations in South Africa suggest, once again, that the higher fiber-containing diet of the latter leads to a much lower rate of this disease. Similarly, war-time observations in Europe, when white bread was scarce in places occupied by

Germany, indicate a close relationship between fiber intake and incidence of appendicitis. Apparently even a small increase in fiber intake was found to have a marked lowering effect in this regard. Children in institutions where the diets were only marginally higher in vegetables and other fiber sources than the diets of children living at home had a lower incidence of appendicitis.

Hemorrhoids refer to a condition in which the veins around the anus or lower rectum are swollen and inflamed as a result of straining to defecate. It is estimated that half the U.S. population experiences hemorrhoids by age 50. As with the other gastrointestinal disorders mentioned before, hemorrhoids can be prevented by eating a high fiber diet and drinking several glasses of water a day, a regimen that leads to soft stools that will pass easily without requiring undue pressure and straining.

CHAPTER 6
Health-related Functions of Fiber-Colon and Breast Cancer

Once again Burkitt, the British surgeon who returned to England after a long stay of service in Africa, suggested firmly that colon cancer was related to the low fiber diets of European and American populations. He was joined in this assessment by other researchers who carried out epidemiological surveys. The main thesis put forth by Burkitt was that a low fiber diet led to prolonged stay of fecal matter in the colon permitting the bacterial flora to metabolize compounds such as bile acids and leading to the formation of carcinogens. Tempting and logical as this hypothesis is, the evidence of a correlation between fiber intake and cancer of the colon is mixed. The concentration of bile acids in the feces is well correlated with the amount of dietary *fat* consumed. It is possible that a relationship between dietary fiber and colon cancer is related to the cholesterol-lowering properties of certain fibers. This is so because it has been observed that people on a low fiber diet had a greater proportion of bacterial metabolites of cholesterol in their feces than did vegetarians who presumably consumed a relatively high fiber diet. It would thus appear that a high fiber diet can be helpful in reducing colon cancer risk through its linkage to cholesterol metabolism. Interestingly, however, the soluble fibers such as pectin and guar gum that seriously lower blood cholesterol (see Chapter 3), are not the ones that have been shown to influence colon cancer. Instead, it is insoluble fibers such as wheat bran and cellulose that seem to be effective.

The insoluble fibers have been shown particularly effective in preventing experimentally induced colon cancer in animals. There are different cancer-causing chemicals that can be fed, injected or instilled into the rectum. In these animal models of colon cancer the inclusion of insoluble fiber in the diet has been generally successful in preventing the disease.

The results of epidemiological observational studies have been mixed. A large European Prospective

Investigation into Cancer and Nutrition found that a higher fiber intake "was associated with an estimated 25% reduction in risk for large bowel cancer." On the other hand, in a large U.S. study, the Polyp Prevention Trial, the effect of an increased fiber and reduced fat diet showed no beneficial effects on the recurrence of polyps. Then, again, a study in Japan found "a decreasing risk of colon cancer with increasing intakes of calcium and insoluble dietary fiber." Researchers at the Arizona Cancer Center in Tucson have recently reexamined the results of the Polyp Prevention Trial just mentioned, as well as another, the Wheat Bran Fiber Trial, and found that there were significant differences in response between men and women: men showed strong decreased risk from fiber whereas the women did not. The investigators suggest that this sex difference in response could well explain the mixed epidemiological responses that have been reported for the relationship between fiber consumption and colon cancer.

Finally, it is interesting to note that recent studies have suggested that a possible contributing factor to the beneficial effects of fiber might be derived from the "fermentation" that fibers can undergo in the colon under the influence of the bacterial flora that exists there and that produces a fatty acid called butyric acid (the fatty acid found in milk fat from which the name butter is derived). Researchers at the University of Texas Medical Branch in Galveston have suggested "a novel molecular mechanism that may explain in part the beneficial effects of dietary fiber in decreasing the risk of colon cancer."

Several important studies have recently been reported that indicated significant beneficial effects from a high fiber diet in relation to breast cancer. In the UK(United Kingdom) Women's Cohort Study with a wide range of exposure to dietary fiber intake, it was concluded that "in pre-menopausal women, total fibre is protective against breast cancer, in particular, fibre from cereals and possibly fruit."

In a study carried out at the University of California, Los Angeles, it was found "that a very-low-fat, high-fiber diet combined with daily exercise results in major reductions in risk factors for breast cancer (even) while subjects remained overweight /obese."

Yet another study, this one from California State University, assessed the relationship between survival after breast cancer diagnosis and dietary fiber, fat, and other nutrients. The researchers suggested that "reduced dietary fat and increased fiber, vegetable, fruit and other nutrients associated with a plant-based high-fiber diet improves overall survival in post-menopausal women after breast cancer diagnosis."

On the other hand, results just reported from The Women's Healthy Eating and Living Study, showed no reduced additional breast cancer events or mortality. In this study 1537 women were on a high vegetable, fruit and fiber diet (30 grams/day). 1551 women were in the comparison group that received USDA healthy food information but did not essentially change their eating habits over the 7.3 year study. All women in both diet treatment groups had been diagnosed with early stage breast cancer; they ranged in age from 18 to 70 years with the average age 53. Despite the large differences in intakes of fruit, vegetables and fiber and a decreased intake also in fat in the high-fiber group, there were no indications of benefit from the diet treatment on additional breast cancer events or mortality. About 10% of women in both diet programs died during the 7-year study, most of them from breast cancer.

An experiment carried out at the Lombardi Cancer Center at Georgetown University in rats involved the feeding of pregnant rat dams (females) diets containing 6% fiber from cellulose, oat, whole wheat or defatted flax flour. The offspring were given a cancer-inducing drug (7,12 dimethylbenz[a]anthracene) at the age of 50 days and the incidence of breast tumors was assessed thereafter. The offspring from mothers fed whole wheat flour had a reduced tumor incidence while the offspring from mothers given defatted flax flour had an increased incidence. By investigating various metabolic measurements, the researchers were able to conclude that the whole wheat dietary exposure appeared to have improved DNA damage repair mechanisms.

A 7-year study carried out by the National Institutes of Health in cooperation with AARP and published in September 2009, looked at the relationship between dietary fiber intake and breast cancer in 185,598 postmenopausal women. The researchers found a significant 13% decrease in the incidence of breast cancer in those women who had a high intake of soluble, but not insoluble fiber. This observation was not modified or altered by changes in fat intake. Since this was an epidemiological study, it is difficult to be certain that fiber alone was the responsible substance accounting for the reduced breast cancer incidence. For instance, in January 2009, Lee et al. published the results of another epidemiological study that included 73,223 Chinese women and looked at the incidence of breast cancer risk in relation to soy food intake. The study provided "strong evidence for a protective effect of soy food intake against premenopausal breast cancer." The efficacy of soy was attributed to its isoflavone content, a substance that was not mentioned and probably not measured in the NIH study mentioned previously.

CHAPTER 7
Health-related Functions of Fiber-Obesity and Weight Maintenance

The biggest public health scourge in the U.S. is the high incidence of obesity among both adults and teenagers. While there are several contributing factors to this serious problem, including lack of an adequate amount of activity by a large segment of the population, the diet, both qualitatively and quantitatively, certainly plays a most important role. This brings us back to the considerations outlined in Chapter 1. A diet low in fiber and usually high in fat and caloric density does not provide the satiety of a high fiber diet that is low in fat and caloric density. Eating fast-food diets of the former variety can be and often is a major culprit in leading people astray to a life of being overweight. Time Magazine recently ran a major article on appetite and how to control it (June 11, 2007). The first of the four recommendations offered to curb appetite before cravings start, is to eat high fiber foods that "stimulate appetite suppressing hormones and make you feel full."

One of the most misleading ways to help lose weight is to opt for a special "diet." Psychologically that's a poor approach because we are so programmed as to appreciate a routine and sticking with the types of food that we are generally used to eating. Switching to a very different pattern of foods is difficult and leads to feelings of deprivation and even withdrawal. If I am told today that tomorrow I am not to eat at all I begin to feel hungry right away. If, on the other hand, I don't eat tomorrow because I am very busy I can easily forego a meal or two without the slightest difficulty.

Instead of going on a "diet" to lose weight, it is much better to stick to the foods one is used to eating, but to cut back on the amounts and to make small changes so as to lower the fat content and increase the fiber content. Most of us engage in a very imbalanced type of food intake: we eat a very small breakfast, a medium-sized lunch and then gorge ourselves on an outsized dinner. With television occupying much of our late evening pastime, we often end up eating additional food between dinner and retiring for the night. This type of eating schedule is conducive to putting on extra, unwanted pounds. The oversized dinner meal leads to what a famous nutritionist (H.H.Mitchell, University of Illinois) termed "the metabolism of plethora." This is a mode of metabolic activity in which the normal body's machinery becomes overwhelmed with nutrients, more than can be handled at the time, and this leads to the conversion of the excess carbohydrate and protein to fat, which is stored.

Jane Brody, the New York Times Health and Nutrition Reporter, stated a similar thesis: .."despite my well-known interest in healthful eating, I don't believe in deprivation....And so I adopted a philosophy that I call controlled indulgence. I allowed myself one small treat each day- perhaps two cookies, a thin slice of cake or pie or a few tablespoons of ice cream."

A number of studies have shown that greater eating frequency of smaller meals is more healthful than the ingestion of fewer, larger meals. Dividing up the total daily quantity of food to be consumed into smaller discrete portions has many advantages for overweight people who want to lose weight. By eating more frequently, hunger between meals is diminished. Moreover, this eating habit provides a great opportunity to introduce high fiber foods into the daily menu as in-between snacks. Small portions of dried fruits such as raisins and apricots, nuts, particularly almonds, which are not too high in fat, fresh/raw vegetables including carrots, mushrooms, celery stalks, broccoli florets and radishes among others, are a marvelous choice of low-calorie, high fiber foods. The vegetables can be eaten with a dip made of fat-free cottage cheese or yogurt to which has been added a little minced garlic and chopped onion.

An important life-style habit to adopt is to learn to eat slowly. This can be achieved by putting down all eating utensils between bites. Slowing down the rate of eating helps reach satiety before large portions of food have passed into the stomach. Of course it goes without saying that the amount of calories consumed daily must be reduced. By choosing the regimen outlined this becomes a doable exercise without undue trauma, particularly if there is a substantial substitution of fibrous food, fruit, vegetable, whole grain cereal, for higher calorie foods, particularly fat and refined carbohydrates such as sugar, starch and white flour.

Two more considerations round out a most doable weight reduction program: engaging in a meaningful exercise program several times a week and having a compassionate spouse, or friend available as a crutch for those difficult periods when the weight doesn't seem to want to come off.

Exercise, contrary to the average layman's expectation, does not help burn off many calories. What it does do is it improves one's stamina and speeds up circulation which, in turn, helps get rid of substances in the blood that produce anxiety and depression. The idea of a crutch is one of the important aspects of commercial weight control programs. Such plans offer a crutch in two ways: first, the other clients who frequent the program are in the same boat and they provide a certain level of comfort to the others. Secondly, the counselor, or advisor, is usually someone who has gone through the experience of weight loss previously and is thus sympathetic and understanding of the difficulties faced.

We made mention above that there are periods when the weight doesn't seem to want to change despite one's Herculean efforts to reduce one's calorie intake. One handicap that is faced when reducing one's food intake is that the body machinery becomes more efficient. This is a built-in evolutionary phenomenon going way back in human history to the days when man had to scrounge for scarce food resources and often faced severe shortages. This led to the survival of those who were more efficient in calorie utilization on a reduced intake. Another finding related to the difficulties experienced by obese people who attempt to lose weight is the frustration encountered, especially at the beginning, when the weight does not want to budge despite much lower food intake and exercise. This problem is transitory and related to a readjustment in the water and fat stores of the body. As fat stores begin to diminish, they initially are replaced by water until this body composition alteration gives way to a reduction in both fat and the water that had replaced it. Thus, patience and, therefore, an understanding spouse or friend can make all the difference in helping to weather this frustrating experience during a well-coordinated weight loss program.

Many, perhaps most, individuals who suffer from obesity find the weight loss program to reach a desirable goal less difficult than the steps that must be taken to maintain that weight. Here we come back to a formula that underlies so much in our harried, busy modern world: adopting a healthful life-style that includes exercise, adequate sleep, carefully controlled food portions and last, but by no means least, a high intake of fiber from fruits, vegetables, whole grain cereals and perhaps from a good fiber supplement as well. The formerly obese person has got to adopt permanently such a life-style to avoid the yo-yo effect experienced by a large percentage of obese people.

In a carefully conducted six-month trial with 52 obese patients, the value of a fiber supplement was strongly confirmed. All patients were given the same reduced calorie diet, but one group was given, in addition a supplement of 7 grams daily of a mixture of beet, barley and citrus fiber. The fiber-treated group lost 12 lbs over the experimental period compared to a weight loss of only 6.6 lbs for the low-fiber group. In the high-fiber group hunger feelings were significantly reduced, whereas on the low-fiber diet the patients experienced a significant increase in hunger pangs.

In another study, overweight college students were given a low-calorie, fiber-enriched bread compared to regular bread as an adjunct to their other food intake. Those consuming the high-fiber bread lost 19 lbs in 8 weeks compared to a loss of 14 lbs on the low-fiber diet. It was conjectured that the high fiber bread was very effective in controlling hunger pangs thus contributing to a lower intake of other foods.

A study with adolescents carried out in Brazil showed that a dietary fiber intake below the recommended level "was associated with being overweight among those students attending public schooling." In this study the consumption of beans as a fiber source was particularly effective in preventing overweight status when the beans were consumed at least 4 times a week.

From Korea we have a report that Goami No. 2 rice which is high in fiber, was very beneficial in significantly lowering body weight, triglycerides, total and low-density cholesterol of obese subjects.

In yet another study, this one from Spain, involving 5000 men and 6600 women there was a significant inverse relationship between total fiber intake and body weight gain over a 5- year period. Among the men there was also a high correlation between weight gain and fruit/vegetable intake; this relationship was not noted in the women.

A survey of almost 18,000 male physicians free of heart disease, diabetes and cancer at the start of the study in 1982, showed a strong inverse relationship between weight-gain and breakfast cereal intake. "Over 8 and 13 years follow-up, respectively, men who consumed breakfast cereal, regardless of type, consistently weighed less than those who consumed breakfast cereal less often (statistically significant p=0.01). Compared with those men who rarely ate breakfast cereal, those who ate one serving/day were 22 and 12% less likely to become overweight during the 8- and 13- year follow-up."

Researchers at the University of Toronto reported interesting results from the ingestion of a high-fiber cereal meal (33 grams insoluble fiber) by healthy young men. In comparison to the consumption of a low-fiber cereal meal, the high-fiber cereal reduced appetite, lowered food intake and prevented blood sugar from rising in response to a meal consumed 75 minutes after the low- or high-fiber cereal intake. The high-and low-fiber diets were equalized as to carbohydrate and total calorie content so that the results observed could legitimately by ascribed to the efficacy of the insoluble fiber.

In a recent follow-up study from the same group the researchers reported that the consumption of a high, insoluble- fiber vs a low, insoluble fiber cereal con-sumed at breakfast was not compensated for by a higher calorie intake at lunch. The high-fiber cereal increased satiety, and plasma glucose was lower both before and immediately after lunch and total calorie consumption for breakfast and lunch was significantly lower with the high-fiber breakfast cereal.

Several Harvard Medical School related groups, in conjunction with Louisiana State University and the National Heart Lung and Blood Institute compared 4 diets over 2 years as to their weight-reducing properties in 811 overweight adults. Two diets were low in fat, two high in fat and within each fat level either a normal or a high protein intake was studied. All diets supplied 20 % of fiber and the results showed that all 4 diets were about equal in promoting weight loss, and improving markers for better health such as better fasting insulin levels and reduced blood lipid risk factors (LDL cholesterol, triglycerides).

CHAPTER 8
Health-related Functions of Fiber- as a Detoxifying Agent

We have already mentioned that certain fibers have great adsorbing properties that lead to the prevention of cholesterol and bile acid absorption in the digestive tract.   Derivatives of cellulose are often used to purify chemical compounds.   Scientists at Loma Linda and Southern California University have found that certain fibers are effective in protecting against the toxic effects of certain drugs and of additives found in food. It is possible that these protective effects are only noted when people on low fiber diets express concern about medical conditions not observed at all in individuals consuming high fiber diets.

Benjamin Ershoff from the Institute for Nutritional Studies in Culver City, California has reported beneficial effects from fiber that counteracted the toxic effects of several chemicals. For instance, he showed that psyllium seed powder, carrot root powder, alfalfa leaf meal and wheat bran counteracted the toxic effects of high doses of the food colors FD&C Yellow No.5 and FD&C Yellow No.6. Cellulose had little or no protective effect nor did the addition of known nutrients show any amelioration of toxic effects. He also observed that dietary fiber protected against toxic doses of the sweetener cyclamate and against Tween 60 (a detergent).

Indian scientists have reported a protective effect of fiber, particularly of pectin, against the toxic effects of an organophosphorus insecticide, pirimiphos-methyl.

Most recently, scientists in Germany reported that dietary fiber from wheat bran protected human colon cells from the toxic effects of 4-hydroxynonenal and hydrogen peroxide. These workers claimed that the protective effect is due to the fermentation of the fiber by gut microorganisms to yield short chain fatty acids that inhibit the growth of tumor cells and also induce the enzymes glutathione S-transferases.

CHAPTER 9
Dietary Calorie Restriction, Longevity and Fiber

In 1935, Clive McKay was among the first to seriously study the effect of food restriction on growth, health pattern and longevity. It is interesting to note the distortions and conjectures that have occurred over time in interpreting these early studies. For instance, in a recent review it was stated that McKay had done the studies in mice when in fact they were carried out in white laboratory rats. Many later descriptions of these studies have assigned a value to the food restriction of 30-40%. We have been unable to confirm these figures since McKay and coworkers do not state food consumption values in their publications.

McKay and his associates reported that the rats that were food-restricted lived significantly longer than those that were not restricted, that fewer rats in the restricted groups had serious respiratory failures and that the incidence of tumors was also much lower in the food restricted rats.

The next serious study of food/calorie restriction in animals was reported from our laboratory in 1963. We used day-old cockerels as the experimental animals since birds develop serious atherosclerosis quite spontaneously with advancing age, even on diets devoid of high fat and cholesterol. One group of cockerels was allowed to eat to appetite while a second group was given 80% of the food that the controls consumed at the same body weight. The experiment was completed after 37 months but periodically birds from both treatment groups were killed and examined for blood cholesterol and aortic atherosclerosis. There was a profound difference in mortality between the two groups: fully three times as many cockerels from the fully-fed control group had died compared with the birds on the food-restricted regimen. There was also significantly less atherosclerosis in the birds on the restricted calorie intake. The calorie-restricted birds looked much peppier with bright red combs than the controls which had droopy, whitish combs and looked "old."

Since the 1970's many more species have been studied in relation to calorie restriction and their longevity. Among them are hamsters, fish, fruit flies, yeast, monkeys and primates.

Two studies authored by Rajindar S. Sohal from the University of Southern California have claimed that the phenomenon of life extension through calorie restriction is NOT true for all species or even all strains within a species. Sohal and associates have reported that the common housefly, Musca domestica, on a calorie-restricted diet, may actually live less long than on an unrestricted diet. They have also reported that a strain of mice, DBA/2, unlike C57BL/6 and B6D2F, does not live longer on a restricted calorie intake. The housefly study was carried out with fully mature, older insects and did best on an unrestricted, all sugar (sucrose) diet. This suggests that the efficacy of calorie restriction is related to the phase of development and growth and may not apply to a post-growth phase where metabolism is essentially one of maintenance only. The DBA/2 strain of mice is smaller than the other two strains and there may also be an explanation related to its growth pattern that explains the results obtained by Sohal and coworkers.

Much progress has also been made in discovering why calorie restriction leads to an extension of life and to a reduction in the rate of certain diseases such as cancer and heart disease.

Dr. Masoro from the University of Texas in San Antonio has formulated a "unifying" theory that attempts to explain the anti-aging effects of calorie restriction. According to this theory, aging "is primarily the result of the accumulation of unrepaired damage due to long-term intrinsic (internal) and extrinsic (external) stressors." To protect against these stressors different mechanisms have evolved. These include antioxidant systems that prevent damage due to "free radicals," x-ray-like waves that damage the cell's operating mechanism; the production of stress response proteins; elevated glucocorticoid levels. All of these stressor responses may work in tandem and help lower blood glucose and insulin levels and body temperature. These markers have all been observed to be associated with increased longevity.

Very recently Libert and colleagues at the Huffington Center on Aging at Baylor College of Medicine reported yet another interesting twist regarding life span extension and reduction: when fruit flies, Drosophila melanogaster, were exposed to nutrient-derived odors, the longevity extending effects of calorie restriction were reversed. On the other hand, a mutation of an odorant receptor extended the flies' life span.

One of the leading researchers on aging is Dr.L. Guarente from MIT. In a recent New York Times interview, Dr. Guarente stated that his research "is not about extending life after people are infirm........The gold standard is health span........If you can extend health span, and you also happen to extend life span, so be it. That's a side benefit."

Guarente and his group have discovered genes that counteract aging. These genes, called *sirtuins*, protect cells from damage during aging.

An additional exciting discovery has recently been published: an antioxidant called *resveratrol* has been shown to extend the life span of several species including mice and to stimulate the body's defense mechanisms in a manner very similar to those observed in calorie-restricted organisms.

So far the scientific evidence that calorie restriction is of benefit in people is still in its infancy. There now exists the Calorie Restriction Optimal Nutrition

Society that was founded as a result of the advocacy by Dr. Roy Walford, a pathologist at the University of California, Los Angeles who published popular diet books on the subject and himself followed a calorie-restricted diet for the last 30 years of his life.

At Washington University in St. Louis, a small group of calorie-restricted people (18, CR) who were members of the Calorie Restriction Optimal Nutrition Society for 6 years, were matched with another group of 18 healthy individuals who had been on a normal diet intake program. The investigators studied risk factors for atherosclerosis, including serum lipids, lipoprotein, plasma glucose and insulin, blood pressure, body composition and carotid artery intima-media thickness. The CR subjects were significantly leaner, serum total cholesterol, low density lipoprotein cholesterol, triglycerides, fasting glucose, fasting insulin, and both systolic and diastolic blood pressure were all markedly lower than in the control group eating a regular, unrestricted diet. The intima media thickness of the aorta was about 40% less in the CR compared with the control subjects. The authors of the study concluded that "based on a range of risk factors, it appears that long-term calorie restriction has a powerful protective effect against atherosclerosis."

In another recent report, patients on a reduced-calorie diet at Louisiana State University had lower insulin levels and body temperature than non-dieters. As pointed out above, both of these measurements appear to be markers for longevity.

It has been known for some time that mammary tumors are reduced in rodents fed a calorie-restricted diet. Recently, it was shown that mammary tumor formation could be prevented in mice by intermittent calorie restriction. A fresh analysis of breast cancer risk in pre-menopausal women, as previously mentioned in CHAPTER 6, in the United Kingdom Women's Cohort Study, found that those consuming a high fiber diet, particularly fiber from cereals and fruit, were at reduced risk compared with women on low fiber diets.

Four prominent gerontologists have recently published a paper asking the government to spend $3 billion annually to achieve the modest goal of delaying the onset of age-related diseases by seven years! A staunch advocate for more dollars to fund aging research is Aubrey de Grey. Some of his opponents think he is a lunatic because he believes that humans could live to 1000, but his call in support of more research and better funding is receiving more careful hearing.

The subject of extending the life span and reducing incidence of disease is so intriguing that innovative studies and interesting results continue to excite us. A group of researchers led by scientists from the Institute of Healthy Aging, University College London, has reported that "deletion of ribosomal S6 protein kinase 1 (S6K1)...... led to increased life span and resistance to age-related pathologies, such as bone, immune,and motor dysfunction and loss of insulin sensitivity." Deleting S6K1, in mice, gave rise to gene expression patterns analogous to those seen in calorie-restriction. Thus pharmacological manipulation of S6K1 might well open a new door to the benefits of a reduced calorie intake.

And in July of 2009 the first results of a 20-year calorie restricted regimen in Rhesus monkeys was published in Science. At this juncture in the study 80% of the calorie-restricted animals survived compared to 50% of the controls. The calorie restriction "delayed the onset of age-associated pathologies. Specifically, calorie restriction reduced the incidents of diabetes, cancer, cardiovascular disease, and brain atrophy." This was the first substantive observation of the beneficial effects of calorie restriction in a primate species!

We end this chapter by coming back to the statement made in the Introduction: materially increasing our consumption of fiber can be a realistic and painless way to reduce/restrict one's calorie intake. There are so many ways to include plenty of fiber in our diet. Most importantly this can be done by making judicious food choices. The tables in the appendix to this book offer assistance in this regard. Furthermore, we have included tasty recipes based also on foods that offer variety and both soluble and insoluble fiber. Finally, there is the opportunity to take advantage of fiber supplements such as Metamucil and SolaGrain.. More on this subject will be presented in the next chapter.

CHAPTER 10
Fiber Supplements

Almost all fiber supplements on the US market today are designed to relieve gastrointestinal problems such as constipation and irritable bowel syndrome. These supplements usually contain only one active fiber source. Among the common products are the following: Benefiber, Konsyl, Grapefruit Fiber, FiberChoice, Citrucel, Metamucil, Acacia Tummy Fiber, Fybogel, Equalactin and Fibercon.

Benefiber, prior to 2006, was said to contain partially hydrolysed guar gum but now some of the products under that name contain wheat dextrin. Two studies reported from Bangladesh tested Benefiber in children with persistent diarrhea. In both instances the Benefiber enhanced the recovery of the children and reduced the duration of diarrhea compared with the control groups. In a report from Switzerland Benefiber was evaluated to determine if it interfered with the absorption of glucose, amino acids or fat in healthy volunteers. The results were negative, no interference with nutrient absorption was shown, nor were insulin release or other pancreatic function affected.

Konsyl and Metamucil are products that contain psyllium as the fiber source. Several studies with psyllium have shown its efficacy in reducing blood cholesterol in hypercholesterolemic individuals, in improving and offering relief in people suffering from irritable bowel syndrome and in significantly improving the metabolic response of type 2 diabetic patients

Psyllium was recently used as a substitute for gluten in bread for celiac disease patients. The acceptance of the psyllium-modified bread was very positive and the modified bread provided less fat and fewer calories.

Grapefruit Fiber is exactly that: a powder made from grapefruit residue that is high in pectin content. As already discussed in Chapter 3, pectin is a potent cholesterol-lowering fiber. It is interesting to note that an electrostatic interaction has been observed between grapefruit pectin and low-density lipoprotein, the material to which the harmful form of cholesterol is attached in the blood stream.

Citrucel contains methylcellulose a substance that is derived from cellulose and has gel-forming attributes that make it suitable as a treatment for constipation. FiberChoice contains inulin, a carbohydrate made up of several simple sugars, mostly fructose, linked together. It is found in many plants and is considered a soluble fiber that is indigestible by human enzymes. Acacia Tummy Fiber is the only pure fiber compound among those listed above. It is made up of gum arabic which is harvested from two species of acacia trees. Equalactin and Fibercon contain as their active ingredient a synthetic compound called calcium polycarbophil. This substance, although not a naturally occurring fiber, has properties that emulate natural fibers. Fybogel contains the bulk-forming fiber ispaghula husk from a plant called Plantago ovata. This substance is very similar to psyllium husks.

Some health-food stores sell pure pectin in capsule or pill form. In pill form pectin is not likely to be effective because it hardens on contact with moisture and then may transit the digestive tract without disintegration.

There are also different brands of wheat-, oat-, and rice bran available in health food stores, some supermarkets and on line. All of these contain indigestible fiber and oat bran is an effective soluble fiber that has been shown to lower blood cholesterol. Wheat bran, while effective, as we pointed out in Chapter 5, in connection with digestive disorders, should be used with some degree of caution. It is relatively high in the organic form of phosphorus called phytin phosphorus. This component of wheat bran binds trace minerals such as iron and zinc and, if used in excess, can produce deficiencies of these trace minerals.

Some thirty years ago I was made aware of another interesting and potentially useful fiber source from barley. The residue from malting in which the starch component of barley is utilized and converted to the sugar maltose, is a high-fiber product that, like oat bran, has been shown in our laboratory to lower blood cholesterol. At the time of our studies fiber was not yet an accepted concept for our human diet. We tried to interest the baking industry to incorporate the barley residue from malting in bread making but with no success. It was only in the mid 1970's when Dr. Burkitt's fame reached Time Magazine that the baking industry woke up to the possibilities of high-fiber baked goods. Barley residue, even after interest in fiber had been aroused, never took off. We discovered that the residue contained a small amount of highly unsaturated fatty acids which, upon storage, became rancid so that the barley residue took on an undesirable flavor and odor.

In 1980 a report from Japan noted the use of Gobo and Konjac fiber in breadmaking. Gobo is a very common food in Japan. It is derived from the root of edible burdock, a thistle-like plant. Konjak is a widely distributed plant in China and Japan and again, the root is used for a variety of food items. The plant and the root must be processed before using because they contain poisons that can be harmful. As stated in Chapter 2, the component of interest in Konjac is glucomannan, a soluble fiber that has cholesterol-lowering properties. In the study from Japan it was observed that a 5 % addition of gobo residue or konjak powder produced very normal breads, little different from breads without these fiber additions. At 10 or 15 % additions, the loaf volume of the breads was reduced.

Inulin and psyllium have been reported to produce more intestinal gas than some of the other fibers. In a carefully conducted study at the University of California, Berkeley, it was found in healthy men that hydrogen gas production increased throughout the day on the high fiber diets while production of methane, the other gas analyzed, was relatively constant throughout the day. Diets high in xylan, a gummy fiber composed of sugar complexes having 5 carbon atoms per molecule, and pectin produced more methane than diets high in cellulose or corn bran. Xylan and pectin also produced more flatus volume than the other two fiber sources, or diets devoid of any of the 4 fibers. Flatus refers to gases in the intestinal tract that are under pressure and often have an odor, usually from a sulfur source. Nitrogen, hydrogen and carbon dioxide, all found as part of intestinal gases, do not have any odor.

Particle size was found to affect transit time of food through the human digestive tract in the case of wheat bran. The coarse bran significantly speeded up food transit time, about 40 hrs, compared to finely ground bran that produced transit times of about 57 hrs. The finely ground bran was much less effective in holding water in the feces, while there were no differences in the digestibility of the food with either type of bran.

The author of this book provided scientific advice in the formulation of a multi-ingredient fiber product called SolaGrain. The rationale for this product was to assist moderately overweight people to lose weight by lowering their calorie intake through increased satiety provided by a fiber supplement and to promote an easier time of maintaining body weight once a desired goal had been reached. The SolaGrain was to be ingested either as part of a food to which it had been added by its manufacturer, for example a bakery product, or in its pure form dissolved in water, juice or soup, in 10 gram quantities three times a day before meals. In this way SolaGrain provides satiety and fullness in the gastrointestinal tract thus making it easier to reduce food portions during breakfast, lunch and dinner. SolaGrain has been successfully incorporated into breads at a level of 16 % and into pizza dough at a level of 25 %. Unlike the reduced loaf volume and other problems encountered in the Japanese study with gobo residue and konjac powder (see above, this Chapter), highly edible and satisfactory breads and pizzas, as well as other products, have been obtained with SolaGrain.

SolaGrain contains soy fiber, oat fiber, psyllium, guar gum, fibersol (an indigestible but water-soluble carbohydrate) and several quality proteins including soy and flax seed. The proteins in SolaGrain provide small but meaningful amounts of essential amino acids and do not add significant amounts of fat to the diet. The flax seed also supplies some fiber as well as antioxidants and contributes a small amount of omega-3-fatty acids.

The protein in SolaGrain provides a balanced mixture of the essential amino acids that are necessary for body protein synthesis. From the perspective of a product designed to assist in health maintenance including weight control, certain essential amino acids, such as tryptophan in particular, serve as the starting material for the body's synthesis of neurotransmitters. It is well established that the neurotransmitter serotonin plays an important role in satiety control in the brain. A craving for carbohydrate and for alcohol has been linked to low concentrations of this neurotransmitter. Thus, providing dietary protein that supplies an adequate amount of tryptophan addresses an issue concerning excessive food intake faced by numerous people who have a weight problem.

It is also well known that weight loss on a low calorie diet or due to starvation does lead to body protein breakdown, even when the person has ample fat stores. It is therefore advisable to include some protein in a low-calorie product, as is the case for SolaGrain, to prevent such body protein loss.

SolaGrain was tested by giving it to a group of 30 female subjects on a weight-loss program for a period of 3 weeks. The group received counseling before starting on the study in which it was emphasized that the objective was to test if it were possible to lose a moderate amount of weight while staying within one's normal eating pattern. A large majority of the participants indicated feeling comfortable, with improved well-being while taking SolaGrain. At the conclusion of the study 4 % lost 8 lbs., 50 % lost from 6 to 7.5 lbs., 31 % lost between 3.5 and 5.25 lbs., 4 % lost 2 lbs., and the rest, or 11 % gained about a lb. or remained the same. Of the original 30 subjects, 28 signed up for another 3-week cycle.

A recent study with SolaGrain was carried out in Germany with 17 women and 10 men all of whom suffered from type 2 diabetes. The subjects ranged in age from 40 to 72 years, were obese, average weight 114 kg, and their Body Mass Index (BMI) was 39.4. Eighteen of the 27 were on insulin, their average total cholesterol was 209 mg/dl and their average HbA1c was 7.6. After 3 months the most important observation was a very significant decrease in the HbA1c, an important measure of diabetes. Weight loss fluctuated among the subjects, some losing as much as 6 to 10 kg while others lost no more than 1 to 4 kg. Cholesterol decreased significantly half-way through the study, but rose again during the latter half. The subjects did not consistently consume the 3 X 10 g daily amount of SolaGrain but on average consumed only about 2 X 10 g. This may explain the initial drop in cholesterol since the subjects adhered more strictly to the prescribed 3 X 10 g intake at the beginning, but during the second half had lowered their intake by one third. Overall, the findings with these severe diabetic, obese patients were very gratifying, enabling several to stop using insulin.

CHAPTER 11
An Everyday, High-Fiber Diet

So what about eating high-fiber diets on an ongoing basis? Aside from deriving various health benefits from fiber as we discussed in the earlier chapters, a high-fiber diet is almost by definition lower in calories than a low-fiber diet. Such a diet is essentially very much a vegetarian diet since fiber, as we defined it previously, is the indigestible residue of plant foods. How healthful is a vegetarian diet and can it sustain us with regards to all the needed nutrients?

Generally, a vegetarian diet is healthful because it is usually much lower in fat, particularly saturated fat and in cholesterol than a diet that includes meat, eggs and dairy products. Moreover, because it is lower in fat, a vegetarian diet also provides fewer calories. Aside from its higher fiber content, a vegetarian diet, if properly balanced by including a variety of different foods, will supply most of the required nutrients in adequate amounts. The nutrients that require some attention on a vegetarian diet are vitamin B_{12} and calcium Vitamin B_{12} can either be taken separately (not a bad idea even on a non-vegetarian diet since vitamin B_{12} and folic acid are important to maintain a normal level of homocysteine, a risk factor for heart disease), or by consuming small amounts of animal products such as fish, eggs or cheese.

With the enormous advance of the food processing industry in recent years we are fortunate to have ready access to dairy products that are free of fat and cholesterol, yet are good sources of calcium. Fat-free milk, yogurt, cream cheese, cottage cheese and sour cream are all easily available in every supermarket. Turkey and chicken meat is also relatively low in fat and cold-cuts prepared from these poultry products are generally nutritious as well. Eggs present a problem because most of the vitamins are found in the yolk which also contains all the fat and cholesterol. Nevertheless, an egg white omelet with fresh mushrooms, peppers and onions can be very tasty and supplies excellent protein quality in addition to the fiber from the vegetables. Last, but certainly not least, fish is the most easily available source of omega-3-fatty acids. There are many excellent, low-fat fish around including Talapia, Flounder, Sole, Halibut and Haddock among others.

There are other benefits that may be derived from selecting a high-fiber, fruit, vegetable and grain diet as part of one's daily food intake. One such benefit is the presence of potent antioxidants in many fruits and vegetables. Red grapes and pomegranates are rich in resveratrol, an antioxidant that has recently been shown to extend the lifespan of mice as mentioned in Chapter 8. Blueberries and cranberries contain other antioxidants that add to our well-being and have been shown to be clinically potent against urinary tract infections. Tomatoes, guava and pink grapefruit contain an antioxidant called lycopene that has been shown to protect against prostate cancer. A number of foods including broccoli, green peas, honeydew melon, kale and kiwi contain another antioxidant called lutein that appears to offer potent protection against macular degeneration, a very serious eye disease. Vegetables such as broccoli, cauliflower and Brussels sprouts contain a substance, glucoraphanin, that is converted upon ingestion into sulforaphane, an anticancer compound. Garlic, leeks and onions contain allicin, a substance that is believed to reduce cancer risk and enhance infection defenses. Cherries have been shown to promote a decrease in blood urate levels, a metabolite that plays an important role in gout. Thus, cherries or cherry juice have considerable efficacy in reducing gout-related inflammation. These are but a few of many examples of useful components present in plant foods that are not directly nutrients, yet possess properties that aid and assist in healthful living.

Two additional pieces of information need to be considered in relation to these beneficial constituents of plant foods: there also exist harmful chemicals in many foods that can damage our health if eaten in large quantities. One such compound, solanine, is present in vegetables of the nightshade family that includes potatoes, tomatoes, eggplants and peppers. We consume these vegetables with great regularity but generally in moderate amounts so that no harm comes to us. On the other hand, some years ago a variety of potatoes was developed in Canada that would thrive under short summer conditions in the far north of the country. When finally ready for marketing, it was discovered that this variety had a much higher solanine concentration than ordinary varieties and might make people sick; it had to be withdrawn from use.   Other potentially harmful chemicals include anti-thyroid compounds that affect the proper functioning of the thyroid gland and the body's metabolic activity. Such substances are present in cabbage, broccoli, turnips and cauliflower.

It is clear from this short presentation that we must at all times be moderate in consuming the different foods we eat. On one hand we want to take advantage of the beneficial components and at the same time we must beware of not ingesting too much of some of the harmful constituents that are likewise present in our food supply. The way to achieve both is to follow a "balanced diet" eating program. A balanced diet is very simple to follow: eat a large variety of different foods, all of them in moderation.

As mentioned earlier when we discussed the various health benefits of fiber, it has been shown time and again that a diet that provides certain compounds from food rather than as pure supplements are often more efficacious, particularly in epidemiological studies with human subjects. Furthermore, since foods rich in fiber are often the same ones that also supply antioxidants and the array of other biologically active substances, a word of caution may be advisable in ascribing all the benefits from a given dietary regime to fiber alone. Nevertheless, when we add the values of the other plant substances we have mentioned to those of fiber, the main theme of this book, we have, I believe, a very strong case for a diet high in fruits, cereals and vegetables. In the appendix you will find some great and tasty recipes that combine lots of vegetables with low-fat animal products. Gourmet eating can include fiber-rich foods!

APPENDIX

Comprehensive Table of Fiber Content of Foods

Source: Journal of Human Nutrition 30:303-313, 1976.
A Guide to calculating intakes of dietary fibre.
Southgate, et al.

Dietary fibre in some vegetables (g/100g edible portion)

	Total dietary fibre	Non-cellulosic polysaccharides	Cellulose	Lignin
Leafy vegetables				
Broccoli tops (boiled)	4.10	2.92	0.85	0.03
Brussels sprouts (boiled)	2.86	1.99	0.80	0.07
Cabbage (boiled)	2.83	1.76	0.69	0.38
Cauliflower (boiled)	1.80	0.67	1.13	Tr
Lettuce (raw)	1.53	0.47	1.06	Tr
Onions (raw)	2.10	1.55	0.55	Tr
Legumes				
Beans, baked (canned)	7.27	5.67	1.41	0.19
Beans runner (boiled)	3.35	1.85	1.29	0.21
Peas, frozen (raw)	7.75	5.48	2.09	0.18
Peas, garden (canned)*	6.28	3.80	2.47	0.01
Peas, processed (canned)*	7.85	5.20	2.30	0.35
Root vegetables				
Carrots, young (boiled)	3.70	2.22	1.48	Tr
Parsnips (raw)	4.90	3.77	1.13	Tr
Swedes (raw)	2.40	1.61	0.79	Tr
Turnips (raw)	2.20	1.50	0.70	Tr

	Total dietary fibre	Non-cellulosic polysaccharides	Cellulose	Lignin
Potato				
Main crop (raw)	3.51	2.49	1.02	Tr
Chips (fried)	3.20	2.05	1.12	0.03
Crisps	11.9	10.6	1.07	0.32
Canned*	2.51	2.23	0.28	Tr
Peppers (cooked)	0.93	0.59	0.24	Tr
Tomato (fresh)	1.40	0.65	0.45	0.30
Tomato (canned)*	0.85	0.45	0.37	0.03
Sweetcorn (cooked)	4.74	4.31	0.31	0.12
Sweetcorn (canned)*	5.69	4.97	0.64	0.08

* Drained

Dietary fibre in some fruit and nuts (g/100g edible portion)

	Total dietary fibre	Non-cellulosic polysaccharides	Cellulose	Lignin
Fruits				
Apples (flesh only)	1.42	0.94	0.48	0.01
Apples (peel only)	3.71	2.21	1.01	0.49
Bananas	1.75	1.12	0.37	0.26
Cherries (flesh & skin)	1.24	0.92	0.25	0.07
Grapefruit (canned)*	0.44	0.34	0.04	0.55
Guavas (canned)*	3.64	1.67	1.17	0.80
Mandarin oranges (canned) *	0.29	0.22	0.04	0.03
Mangoes (canned)*	1.00	0.65	0.32	0.03
Peaches (flesh & skin)	2.28	1.46	0.20	0.62
Pears (flesh only)	2.44	1.32	0.67	0.45
Pears (peal only)	8.59	3.72	2.18	2.67
Plums (flesh and skin)	1.52	0.99	0.23	0.30
Rhubarb (raw)	1.78	0.93	0.70	0.15
Strawberries (raw)	2.12	0.98	0.33	0.81
Strawberries (canned)*	1.00	0.48	0.20	0.33
Sultanas	4.40	2.40	0.83	1.17
Nuts				
Brazils	7.73	3.60	2.17	1.96
Peanuts	9.30	6.40	1.69	1.21

* Fruit & syrup

Dietary fibre in wheat flours and bread (g/100g)

	Total dietary fibre	Non-cellulosic polysaccharides	Cellulose	Lignin
Flours				
White, breadmaking	3.15	2.52	0.60	0.03
Brown	7.87	5.70	1.42	0.75
Wholemeal	9.51	6.25	2.46	0.80
Bran	44.0	32.7	8.05	3.23

	Total dietary fibre	Non-cellulosic polysaccharides	Cellulose	Lignin
Breads				
White	2.72	2.01	0.71	Tr
Brown	5.11	3.63	1.33	0.15
Hovis	4.54	2.99	1.01	0.04
Wholemeal	8.50	5.95	1.31	1.24

* Expressed as the sum of the component monosaccarides
+ Expressed as glucose

Dietary fibre in some breakfast cereals (g/100g)

	Total dietary fibre	Non-cellulosic polysaccharides	Cellulose	Lignin
All-bran	26.7	17.82	6.01	2.88
Cornflakes	11.0	7.26	2.42	1.32
Grapenuts	7.00	5.14	1.28	0.58
Readibrek	7.60	5.39	0.99	1.22
Rice Krispies	4.47	3.47	0.78	0.22
Puffed Wheat	15.41	10.35	2.59	2.47
Sugar Puffs	6.08	4.00	0.99	1.09
Shredded Wheat	12.26	8.79	2.63	0.84
Special K	5.45	3.68	0.72	1.05
Swiss breakfast (mixed brands)	7.41	5.31	1.36	0.74
Weetabix	12.72	9.18	2.35	1.19

* Expressed as the sum of the component monosaccarides
** Expressed as glucose
+ This value may include heat induced artefacts analysing as lignin

Dietary fibre in some biscuits (g/100g)

	Total dietary fibre	Non-cellulosic polysaccharides	Cellulose	Lignin
Chocolate digestive (1/2 coated)	3.50	2.13	0.59	0.78
Chocolate (fully coated)	3.09	1.36	0.42	1.31
Crispbread, rye	11.73	8.33	1.66	1.74
Crispbread, wheat	4.83	3.34	0.94	0.55
Ginger biscuits	1.99	1.45	0.30	0.24
Matzo	3.85	2.72	0.70	0.43
Oatcakes	4.00	3.16	0.40	0.44
Semi-sweet	2.31	1.76	0.33	0.22
Short-sweet	1.66	1.42	0.11	0.13
Wafers (filled)	1.62	1.08	0.47	0.07

INDEX

Recipes
Main Dishes

Chinese-Style Chicken Cutlets

1/4 cup corn syrup
1/4 cup water
1 tablespoon starch
1 clove garlic minced
2 tablespoons low-sodium
  soy sauce
2 tablespoons sherry
1/4 tablespoon corn oil

2 whole chicken breasts,
  boned, skinned, cut in
  1/2-inch pieces
2 tomatoes, cut in wedges
1 green pepper, cut in 1/2-
  inch pieces
1 package frozen Chinese
  peapods (or 1/2 pound
  fresh snow peas)

Place corn syrup, water, starch, garlic, soy source, sherry and ginger in small bowl and stir together. Heat olive oil over medium-high heat in a large skillet. Add chicken pieces and cook, stirring occasionally, about 3 minutes or until done. Stir tomatoes, green pepper, and peapods, then add corn syrup mixture from bowl. Bring to boil, stirring constantly, and continue to boil for one minute.

4 servings
34 mg cholesterol, 268 Calories/serving.

Veal Marsala

1-1/2 pounds thinly cut,
   trimmed veal
1 clove finely chopped or
   pressed garlic
2 tablespoons parsley

1 tablespoon basil
1 small can or 3/4 pound
   fresh sliced mushrooms
1/2 cup Marsala wine

Preheat oven to 325°F. Cut veal into 3/4–1-inch squares. Lightly brown in skillet pregreased with nonstick vegetable cooking spray. Add all other ingredients, cover, and cook in oven for about 40-50 minutes.

6 servings
104 mg cholesterol, 277 Calories/serving.

Poached Sole Julienne

1-1/2 pounds of filets of sole
2 cups diced cherry tomatoes
1/2 zucchini, julienned
   (cut lengthwise in strips)

2 carrots, julienned
2 celery stalks, julienned
1 cup dry white wine
low-sodium salt to taste

Preheat oven to 350°F. Place filets in baking dish and cover with diced tomatoes, zucchini, carrots, and celery. Pour in wine. Cover and bake for 20-30 minutes or until tender.

4 servings
138 mg cholesterol, 277 Calories/serving.

Bean Cassoulet

6 cups water
1-1/2 pounds Navy beans
Low-sodium salt to taste
1/4 teaspoon pepper
2 cans low-sodium
   condensed chicken broth
2 tablespoons corn oil
2 tablespoon bacon bits
8 pieces of chicken
4 quartered carrots
3 halved onions

4 whole cloves
2 bay leaves
3 cloves crushed garlic
1/2 cup coarsely chopped
   celery leaves
1/2 teaspoon thyme
1 teaspoon marjoram
1 teaspoon sage
1 can peeled tomatoes
1 pound chicken hot dogs
chopped parsely

Boil 6 cups of water in large kettle. Add beans, salt and pepper. Cook for 2 minutes. Remove from heat, cover, and let soak for 1 hour. Add broth. Return to boil, cover and cook for one more hour. Brown chicken parts in skillet greased with corn oil. In a 6-quart casserole, mix beans, cooking liquid, bacon bits, chicken parts, vegetables, herbs, and undrained tomatoes. Cover and bake in oven at 350°F for 1 hour. Add chicken hot dogs cut diagonally in pieces. Bake for another 20–30 minutes or until beans are tender. Garnish with chopped parsley.

8 servings
68 mg cholesterol, 599 Calories/serving.

Chicken-Stuffed Peppers

6 large green peppers

6 medium-size tomatoes, or 1-pound, 12-ounce can

2 cups cut-up cooked chicken

2 cups chopped zucchini

1/4 cup chopped onion

1 tablespoon chopped parsely

2 tablespoons chopped red pepper

1/4 teaspoon low-sodium salt

1/4 teaspoon oregano

1/8 teaspoon ground black pepper

1 cup shredded bran cereal

1/3 cup packaged quick rice

1 15-ounce can tomato sauce

Cut off tops of green peppers and remove seeds. Cook in large pan of boiling water for 5 minutes, drain, and set aside. Prepare stuffing: Chop tomatoes, saving the liquid; in a bowl, combine tomato, tomato liquid, and all remaining ingredients except tomato sauce. Spoon stuffing into green peppers and place peppers in a shallow baking dish, adding enough water to cover bottom. Bake at 350°F for about 30 minutes, or until peppers are just tender. Heat tomato sauce in a small saucepan and pour over peppers when ready to serve.

6 servings
18 mg cholesterol, 175 Calories/serving.

Babootie: African Curried Stew

2 tablespoons corn oil
4 onions, 1 chopped very
fine, 3 coarsely chopped
1 clove garlic, chopped fine
3/4 pound ground veal
1/2 cup rolled oats
2 teaspoons cinnamon
1 pound canned tomatoes,
preferably in tomato puree
2–3 tablespoons curry
powder
2 tablespoons vinegar
2 slightly overripe bananas
sliced

1/2 cup raisins or currants
1 stalk celery with leaves
chopped
2 tart apples, unpeeled,
cored, chopped fine
2 dried apricots, chopped
fine (or 2 fresh or canned
apricots in light syrup,
chopped)
1/4 cup almonds, slivered or
whole (skins on)
tomato juice or water for
thinning
1/4 cup parsely, chopped fine
for garnish

Heat corn oil in large skillet. Add 3 coarsely chopped onions and garlic and sauté over low heat. Mix ground veal, finely chopped onion, rolled oats, and cinnamon and shape into 1-inch-diameter meat balls (makes about 25). Add meatballs to onions and sauté gently until meatballs are brown. Add tomatoes with liquid from can, curry powder, and vinegar and bring to boil over medium heat. Add bananas, raisins, celery, most of the apples (reserve some more for garnish), apricots, and almonds. Lower heat and simmer gently, stirring often, for about 20–30 minutes. Thin with tomato juice or water if stew gets very thick. Garnish with chopped apples and parsley. Babootie is excellent served over steamed brown rice.

4–6 servings
48 mg cholesterol, 490 Calories/serving.

Victorious Veal Sauté-Stew

Flower
Sea salt
Pepper, fresh ground
2-1/2 pounds veal cut into
   cubes for stewing
1 teaspoon paprika
1 teaspoon rosemary
1 teaspoon thyme

1 cup vermouth
1/2 cup water
12 small white onions, peeled
4 carrots, scraped and sliced
1/2 cup sliced mushrooms
1/2 cup scallions, chopped
1/2 cup fresh green peas,
   cooked

Mix flour, salt and pepper. Dredge (coat) veal cubes well with mixture and brown on all sides in greased skillet, sprinkling with a little paprika as they cook. Add rosemary, thyme, vermouth, and water, cover, and simmer gently for about 40 minutes. Add white onions and carrots, cover, and simmer again until vegetables are nearly tender and veal is cooked through. For the last few minutes of cooking, add mushrooms and scallions. Finally, add peas with just enough time to be heated before serving. (If the stew is too watery, thicken with all-purpose flour mixed into low-fat yogurt.)

4 servings
121 mg cholesterol, 302 Calories/serving.

Meat Balls á la Seoul with Stir-Fried Vegetables

3/4 pound tofu
(soybean curd)
3/4 pound ground veal
4 scallions, chopped fine
1 clove garlic, chopped fine
1 tablespoon toasted sesame
seeds
1/2 teaspoon sugar
1 tablespoon low-sodium soy
sauce
Dash of cayenne pepper
2 tablespoons pine nuts
4 tablespoons wholw wheat
flower

3 tablespoons sesame oil
2 cups fresh chopped
vegetables for stir
frying–onions, celery,
green peppers, carrots,
bok choy, parsely, romaine
lettuce, or snow peas in a
combination of your
choice
1 tablespoon sherry
Chopped parsely for garnish

In a bowl, mix tofu, ground veal, scallions, garlic, sesame seeds, sugar soy sauce, and cayenne pepper. Shape into walnut-size balls and insert two pine nuts in each ball. Roll balls lightly in flour. Heat sesame oil in skillet or wok, add meat balls, five or six at a time, and sauté over high heat until cooked all the way through (about five minutes). Remove and place on paper towels to drain off excess oil.

Stir-fry vegetables in skillet for 3-5 minutes. Add meat balls and sherry and stir-fry for another minute or two to reheat. Serve over steamed brown rice and garnish with sesame seeds or chopped parsley.

4 servings
61 mg cholesterol, 428 Calories/serving.

Sweet-Sour Lentils with Turkey Hot Dogs

2 cups lentils
6 cups low-sodium chicken
   broth
2/3 cup lemon juice

3/4 cup sugar or sugar
   substitute
1 pound turkey hot dogs

Wash and drain lentils. Combine with broth and cook in pressure cooker 20–25 minutes. When lentils are soft, add lemon juice, sugar, and salt. Cook hot dogs separately and, when ready, simmer with lentils for 10 minutes.

5 servings
38 mg cholesterol, 365 Calories/serving.

Side Dishes

Relish Supreme

2 cups cooked brown rice
1 cup canned whole-kernel
   corn
1 cup cooked green peas
1/2 cup minced onions,
   sautéed lightly
1/2 cup red pepper, minced
3 tablespoons chopped
   parsley

1/4 cup corn oil
1/4 cup wine vinegar
1/4 teaspoon low-sodium salt
1/4 teaspoon garlic powder
1/4 teaspoon fresh-ground
   pepper

Combine first six ingredients in a large bowl and mix thoroughly. Add remaining ingredients and toss lightly. Refrigerate until needed.

8 servings
0 mg cholesterol, 149 Calories/serving.

Healthful Fried Rice

4 tablespoons corn oil
5 scallions, cut in 1/2-inch
  lengths
2 cups finely chopped carrots
  and mushrooms
1 tablespoon chopped fresh
  ginger
1 cup cooked, diced breast of
  chicken (without skin)

4 cups cooked cold brown
  rice
1-1/2 tablespoons low-
  sodium soy sauce
2 teaspoons sugar (optional)
2 tablespoons dry sherry
4 egg whites, lightly beaten

Heat 1 tablespoon corn oil in skillet or wok and stir-fry scallions for 1/2 minute. Add chopped carrots, mushrooms, and ginger and stri-fry briefly until tender but still firm. Add chicken, heat through, then remove contents from pan.

Add rest of oil to pan and heat until very hot. Add rice, stirring carefully to avoid lumping. After rice is heated through, add vegetable-chicken mixture and stir, blending in soy sauce, sugar and sherry. Gently fold in egg whites. As soon as they set, remove from heat.

4 servings
28 mg cholesterol, 409 Calories/serving.

Fortifying Hommus

1/2 cup diced onion
2 cloves garlic, minced
1 cup cooked chick peas
   (garbanzos)
3 tablespoons corn or
   safflower oil
2 tablespoons chopped fresh
   spearmint, or 1 tablespoon
   crushed dry mint leaves
   (optional)

1/4 cup tahini (sesame seed
   butter, available in Middle
   Easter or Oriental
   groceries)
1/4 cup lemon juice

In skillet, sauté onion and garlic in 1 tablespoon of oil until slightly soft. Place in blender with all other ingredients, including remaining oil, and blend until smooth. Delicious as a spread for raw vegetable salads or sandwich filling for pita pockets.

4 servings
0 mg cholesterol, 400 Calories/serving.

Quick-Baked Potato Strips

6 potatoes
2-1/2 tablespoons corn oil
1/2 teaspoon paprika

1/8 teaspoon pepper
Low-sodium salt to taste

Preheat oven to 450°F. Wash potatoes and cut lengthwise into strips. Mix oil with spices. Dip potato strips into oil mixture, drain excess oil, and place strips on a baking sheet. Bake for 15 minutes.

10 servings
0 mg cholesterol, 93 Calories/serving.

Sweet and Sour Mélange

1/4 cup corn or safflower oil
2 cups tofu, diced
2 carrots, scraped and thinly
    sliced
1/4 cup scallions, chopped
1 tablespoon cornstarch

1/4 cup low-sodium soy
    sauce
8 cherry tomatoes, quartered
1 9-ounce can crushed
    pineapples, drained
1/2 cup blanched almonds

Heat oil in skillet or wok, then sauté tofu, carrots, and scallions for 3 minutes. Dissolve cornstarch in soy sauce, add to pan, stir, and add tomatoes. Cook for 5 minutes. Add pineapples and almonds and cook for 2 more minutes.

4 servings
0 mg cholesterol, 357 Calories/serving.

Snacks and Appetizers

Almond-Raisin Mix

1 pound freshly shelled
    almonds

3/4 pound seedless raisins or
    currants

Mix together and store in plastic bag in refrigerator.

30 servings
0 mg cholesterol, 123 Calories/serving.

Breakfast Dishes

Granola

5 cups uncooked rolled oats
1 cup sunflower seeds
1 cup sesame seeds
1 cup wheat germ
1 cup wheat bran
1/2 cup nonfat dry milk
  powder
1/2 cup corn oil
1 cup honey

Blend dry ingredients. in a large bowl. In a separate bowl, mix oil and honey. Pour honey-oil mixture over dry ingredients and blend. (if blend is too dry, make and add more of the honey-oil mixture.) Pour blend onto cookie sheet and bake at 300°F for 35–40 minutes. After cooling, store in glass container in refrigerator.

24 servings
Less than 1 mg cholesterol, 194 Calories/serving.

Whole Wheat French Toast

Egg substitute equivalent to
  1 egg
1 tablespoon skim milk
2 slices whole wheat bread
Sugar-cinnamon mixture

Combine egg substitute with skim milk. Soak bread slices in mixture. Brown evenly on both sides in a lightly greased frying pan. Sprinkle with sugar-cinnamon mixture.

2 servings
Less than 1 mg cholesterol, 110 Calories/serving.

Power Pancakes

1/2 cup unbleached flour
1/4 cup rolled oats,
   preferably old-fashioned,
   uncooked
1/2 tablespoon baking
   powder

Pinch of low-sodium salt
1/2 cup skim milk
1/8 cup egg substitute
1 tablespoon vegetable oil

Heat lightly oiled griddle over medium-high gas flames (or pre-heat electric griddle or skillet to 375ºF) Combine dry ingredients in bowl. Add milk, egg substitute, and oil, and stri lightly until dry ingredients are moistened. For each pancake, pour about 1/4 cup batter on hot griddle. Turn when tops are covered with bubbles and edges turn brownish. Turn just once.

6 servings
4 mg cholesterol, 94 Calories/serving.

Soups

Potato Soup

2 leeks
2 onions
2 tablespoons corn oil
5 potatoes, peeled and sliced
4 cups low-sodium chicken
   broth

1 cup low-fat yogurt
1/8 teaspoon pepper
Low-sodium salt to taste

Chop leeks and onions and sauté in corn oil. Add potatoes and chicken broth. Simmer about 15 minutes until potatoes are tender. Put through blender and add yogurt, pepper, and salt.

8 servings
0 mg cholesterol, 149 Calories/serving.

Garlic Soup

3 pressed cloves of fresh
  garlic

Potato soup (see recipe) with
  indicated substitutions

Substitute 3 cloves of garlic for the leeks and onions in potato soup recipe and follow other instructions.

8 servings
0 mg cholesterol, 149 Calories/serving.

Midnight Sun Fruit Soup

1-1/2 quarts water
1 orange with peel, sliced
  thin
1 lemon with peel, sliced
  thin
1/2 cup raisins
1/2 cup diced pineapple,
  fresh or canned
  (unsweetened)
4 tablespoons honey
2 tablespoons tapioca
1/4 teaspoon low-sodium salt
1/2 cup blueberries

1/2 cup diced peaches
  unpeeled
1 cup fresh cherries, pitted
1/2 cup mandarin orange
  sections
2 tablespoons fresh lemon
  juice
1 teaspoon orange extract
1 teaspoon lemon extract
1/2 teaspoon cinnamon
1/2 teaspoon nutmeg
1 cup seedless white grapes

Combine first eight ingredients in large soup kettle and cook 20 minutes. Remove from fire and cool for 10 minutes. Add remaining ingredients, mix thouroughly, and refrigerate. Serve very cold.

8 servings
0 mg cholesterol, 144 Calories/serving.

The Greatest Bean Soup Ever

1 cup minced red onion
1 cup minced celery
1/4 cup corn oil or other vegetable oil
3 cloves garlic, minced
4 quarts water
1/2 cup dried chick peas (garbanzos)
1/2 cup dried lima beans
1/2 cup dried pea beans
1/2 cup dried black beans

2 new potatoes, diced with skin
1/2 diced carrots 1/2 cup barley
1 cup tomato puree
3 tablespoons minced fresh parsely
2 tablespoons minced fresh dill
1 teaspoon oregano
1 teaspoon rosemary
1 teaspoon celery seed

In a large soup kettle, sauté onion and celery in oil until soft. Add remaining ingtedients, cover, and bring to boil. Cook on low flame about 2 hours, or until all beans are tender, stirring occasionally.

8 servings
0 mg cholesterol, 257 Calories/serving.

Dips

Onion Dip

1/2 pint low-fat cottage cheese
1/2 pint low-fat plain yogurt

1 envelope onion soup mix

Mix ingredients thoroughly and refrigerate. Serve with cut-up vegetables (e.g., carrots, celery, broccoli, cauliflower, or mushrooms).

8 servings
0 mg cholesterol, 82 Calories/serving.

Salads

Curried Chicken Calcutta Salad

2 cantaloupes or honeydew
   melons
2 cups chicken breast,
cooked and shredded
1/3 cup no-cholesterol
   mayonnaise (see recipe)
1 tablespoon Dijon mustard

1 tablespoon curry powder
2 cups diced celery
2 cups diced mangos
2 tablespoons sesame seeds
Paprika
Parsely, finely chopped

Cut melons into halves and scoop out centers. Mix shredded chicken, mayonnaise, mustard, curry, celery, mangos, and sesame seeds until uniform. Put mixture in cavities of melon halves. Sprinkle with paprika and garnish with parsley.

4 servings
55 mg cholesterol, 455 Calories/serving.

Tofu Salad

1 package tofu
1 minced onion
1 stalk chopped celery
1 tablespoon wheat germ
2 teaspoons garlic powder

2 tablespoons low-fat plain
   yogurt
1 tablespoon no-cholesteroil
   mayonnaise (see recipe)

Mash and drain tofu and mix with onions, celery, and wheat germ. Sprinkle with garlic powder and add yogurt and mayonnaise. Mix until well blended.

4 servings
55 mg cholesterol, 455 Calories/serving.

Spinach Salad

2 quarts washed and well
  drained spinach leaves
Bacon bits (soy protein)
2 hard-boiled egg whites
  coarsely chopped
5 scallions, chopped
3/4 cup garlic croutons
1/4 cup low-fat plain yogurt

2 teaspoons mustard
1/4 cup lemon juice
1/2 cup cup corn oil
1 tablespoon tarragon vinegar
1/8 teaspoon sugar
Freshly ground black pepper
Dash of low-sodium salt

Tear spinach leaves into small pieces and place in salad bowl. Arrange bacon bits, egg whites, scallions, and croutons over the spinach. Combine all other ingredients and mix well to make dressing. Just before serving, or at the table, pour dressing over salad and toss lightly.

8 servings
0.5 mg cholesterol, 197 Calories/serving.

Egg Plant Salad

1 medium-sized eggplant
2 hard-boiled egg whites
1 teaspoon garlic powder
1/4 teaspoon pepper

1/2 green pepper, diced small
3 tablespoons no-cholesterol
  mayonnaise (see recipe)
Dash of low-sodium salt

Wash eggplant and puncture outer skin in several places with fork. Wrap in heavy aluminum foil and place directly on medium gas flame. Turn occasionally while eggplant softens. When it is completely soft, remove from flame, open foil, and cut in half length-wise. Allow to cool, then scrape softened meat away from skin into a mixing bowl. Make egg whites and combine with eggplant. Add all other ingredients and mix thoroughly.

5 servings
0 mg cholesterol, 32 Calories/serving.

Palace Salad

2 Delicious or Granny Smith apples, chopped but not peeled
1 cup chopped celery
1 11-ounce can mandarin oranges, drained
1 medium firm banana, diced
1/2 cup chopped pecans
1/4 cup no-cholesterol mayonnaise (see recipe)
1/4 cup low-fat plain yogurt
1 tablespoon honey
1 teaspoon Dijon mustard
1/2 teaspoon fresh grated ginger, or 1/4 teaspoon powdered ginger

Mix first five ingredients in a glass salad bowl. Combine the other five for the dressing, pour, on salads, and mix thoroughly. Chill. Serve on a bed of romaine lettuce leaves or watercress.

4 servings
0 mg cholesterol, 358 Calories/serving.

Deserts

Scrumptious Rice Pudding

2 cups cooked brown rice
8 ounces egg substitute
2 cups skim milk
1/4 teaspoon low-sodium salt
1/4 cup brown sugar
1/2 cup raisins or currants

1/2 teaspoon fresh grated
   ginger, or 1/4 teaspoon
   powdered dry ginger
1/2 teaspoon nutmeg
1 teaspoon cinnamon
6 teaspoons maple syrup

Preheat oven to 400°F. Coat 1-1/2-quart casserole with non-stick vegetable cooking spray. In casserole, combine all ingredients except nutmeg, cinnamon, and maple syrup. Sprinkle top generously with nutmeg and cinnamon. Put filled casserole into a slightly larger baking dish or cake pan. Pour boiling water into outer pan to as high a level as possible without spilling water into casserole. Place casserole in its water bath into oven. Bake 1 hour, stirring occasionally to keep rice and raisins (or currants) from settling to the bottom. When liquid has almost all become like custard in texture, turn off oven and leave pudding inside until ready to serve. Serve hot with 1/2-1 teaspoon of maple syrup as topping for each serving.

8 servings
1 mg cholesterol, 153 Calories/serving.

Carrot Delight

1/2 cup sugar
1 cup finely blended carrots
Egg substitute equivalent to
1 egg
1 cup skim milk
1 tablespoon lemon juice

1 teaspoon lemon rind
1/2 cup chopped almonds
2-1/4 cups whole wheat
    flour
2 teaspoons baking soda
1 teaspoon baking powder
1/2 teaspoon low-sodium salt

Preheat oven to 350ºF. In mixing bowl, blend together sugar, carrots, egg substitute, skim milk, lemon juice, and lemon juice, and lemon rind. Add chopped almonds, then flour, baking soda, baking powder, and salt. Stir until well blended. Place batter in 9-inch baking dish pregreased with nonstick vegetable cooking spray and bake for 25–30 minutes.

10 servings
Less than 1 mg cholesterol, 184 Calories/serving.

Johnny Appleseed Cake

3 cups unsweetened apple
    sauce
2 cups rolled oats
2 cups whole wheat flour
1 cup chopped nuts
1/2 cup wheat germ

1/2 cup raisins or currants
1 teaspoon cinnamon
1 teaspoon vanilla extract
1/2 teaspoon allspice
Pinch of low-sodium salt
Confectioners sugar

Mix all ingredients except sugar to form soft, crumbly dough. Press into two 9-inch cake pans, pregreased with nonstick vegetable cooking spray. Bake in medium (350ºF) oven for 50 minutes, or until sides and bottom of cake are brown. Remove from oven and let cool for 10 minutes. Turn out of pans onto rack to cool further. Dust with sugar.

12 servings
0 mg cholesterol, 250 Calories/serving.

Apple-Oat Cake

4–5 tart apples
1/4 cup water
1 cup corn oil
1 cup nut pieces
1 cup raisins or currants
1 cup wheat germ
2 cups rolled oats

2–2-1/2 cups whole wheat
 flour
1/4 teaspoon low-sodium salt
1 teaspoon cinnamon
1/2 teaspoon allspice
1 teaspoon vanilla
1/2 cup dark brown sugar
Confectioners sugar

First make 3 cups applesauce: core and coarsely chop unpeeled apples. Put in saucepan with water. Bring to boil, cover, lower heat, and simmer until pieces are just soft enough to mash. Mix with other ingredients to form soft, crumbly dough. Press into two 9-inch round cake pans, pregreased with nonstick vegetable cooking spray. Bake in medium (350°F) oven for 50 minutes until sides and bottom of cake are brown. Remove from oven and let cool for 10 minutes, then turn out of pan on to rack to cool further. Dust with confectioners sugar..

12 servings
0 mg cholesterol, 520 Calories/serving.

A Shopping List

Dairy Case and Frozen Foods

Egg substitute
Skim milk
Low-fat yogurt
Low-fat cottage cheese
Skim-milk mozzarella, ricotta, farmer, and parmesan cheeses
Corn oil margarine
Tofu (soybean curd)

Tofu frozen dessert (cholesterol and fat-free ice cream)
Orange juice popsicles
Frozen fruit (no sugar or syrup)
Frozen vegetables (no sauces or butter)

Vegetables and Fruits

Enjoy what's in season, but be particularly hospitable to:

Lettuce: romaine, escarole, chicory
Broccoli
Spinach and kale
Peppers (red more nutritious than green)
Tomatoes
Celerty
Onions, all kinds
Mushrooms
Green beans
Green peas
Lima beans

Parsley
Potatoes
Sweet potatoes
Carrots
Cabbage, red and green
Squash, all kinds
Corn
Greens (mustard, dandelion, watercress, arugala)
Apples
Pears
Oranges

Bananas
Lemons
Grapefruit
Grapes
Avacados
Peaches
Apricots
Melons
Berries
Blueberries
Cranberries
Mangos and papayas
Figs and dates
Rhubarb

Hans Fisher was born in Breslau, Germany and left that country to escape the Nazis in May 1939 on the SS St. Louis. The ship traveled to Cuba but was not allowed to discharge its passengers there. Neither the US nor Canada permitted entrance to the 937 refugees. The boat returned to Europe and Fisher and his mother and sister ended up in France. In January 1940, several months after the outbreak of WW II, he was able to leave France and make his way to Cuba where his father had been stranded since January 1939. The family came to the US in February 1941 and settled on a farm in Vineland, NJ. Fisher graduated valedictorian of his high school class. His record earned him a 4-year scholarship to Rutgers University where he obtained a B.S. degree. He followed this with a M.S degree from the U. of Connecticut and finally a Ph.D. in nutritional biochemistry from the University of Illinois in Champaign-Urbana. From 1954-2009 he served on the faculty of Rutgers University, rising through the ranks to Professor II (Distinguished Professor). He started the Department of Nutrition in 1966 and served as its chair for 22 years. He next served as Associate Provost for the Life Sciences. Fisher's research included amino acid metabolism, atherosclerosis and cholesterol, histamine and, carnosine metabolism in relation to wound healing, and tryptophan metabolism in relation to alcoholism and neurotransmitters. He is the author of The Rutgers Guide to Lowering your Cholesterol and over 260 scientific articles in peer-reviewed journals. Fisher and his wife Ruth Hirschberg Fisher have been married for 59 years and have three accomplished children and ten grandchildren

9 780615 348544